say
no
to
placenta
pics

and other hilarious, unsolicited advice for pregnant women

JILLIAN M. PARSONS
WITH ALLISON BAERKEN

Skyhorse Publishing

Skyhorse Publishing books may be purchased in bulk at special discounts for sales promotion, corporate gifts, fund-raising, or educational purposes. Special editions can also be created to specifications. For details, contact the Special Sales Department, Skyhorse Publishing, 307 West 36th Street, 11th Floor, New York, NY 10018 or info@skyhorsepublishing.com.

Skyhorse® and Skyhorse Publishing® are registered trademarks of Skyhorse Publishing, Inc.®, a Delaware corporation.

Visit our website at www.skyhorsepublishing.com.

10 9 8 7 6 5 4 3 2 1

Library of Congress Cataloging-in-Publication Data is available on file.

Cover design by Jane Sheppard and Mona Lin
Cover photo credit: iStockphoto

Print ISBN: 978-1-5107-3372-5
Ebook ISBN: 978-1-5107-3373-2

Printed in the United States of America

DEDICATION

For my parents—as not a "last" but certainly a "ditch" effort
to make up for my teenage years . . . and my twenties
(and for Graham xo)
—Jillian

To Vera, Renée, and Wijnand
—Allison

CONTENTS

FOREWORD FOR MOMS

I swore I'd never become one—but I did, and you might, too. You know, *those* women we all talk about before we have children of our own because of the ridiculous things they sometimes do and say. It can range from the daily clichéd Facebook pictures of their baby, even though nothing has changed from yesterday's identical photo, or criticism that so and so's baby is on formula instead of being breastfed.

But fast-forward to the birth of my daughter. I felt the same compulsion to overshare because I was consumed with motherhood and wanted everyone to feel my joy. Whether I was insisting friends and family to wash their hands before holding her or not being able to leave her for even one night (I still can't!), my stringent regiment could be seen as extreme at times and it caused my friends to roll their eyes.

The truth is, nothing can fully prepare or prevent you from doing the same things I did. At the very least, this book will teach you how to have a sense of humor about the experience of pregnancy—without alienating your friends and family in the process!

—*Allison Baerken, a "Mom"*

FOREWORD FOR NON-MOMS

My wingmen were starting to fail me. Sorry . . . wing-*women* (wing-wo*myn*?). Their disappearance became increasingly evident as I moved through my twenties, and by age thirty I was the only one left in the inner circle buying two-for-one wine on a Monday night (that's *two* bottles for *one* person). It was official—the bottom had completely fallen out of my wild weekends, and I was hard pressed to find anyone who cared or who wasn't too preoccupied to notice. What the hell happened? Where had all the girlfriends gone? I had so many questions, and I didn't have to look far for the answers. Because they literally hadn't "gone" anywhere. They were at home, and they were busy. Busy being, or busy becoming, Moms.

You know, it's really an issue of timing. If someone you knew got knocked up in the throes of adolescence, it was usually a one-off. For many of us, the baby-crazies felt light-years away, even when we came around the bend of twenty-five. I guess I mistakenly presumed we shared the same belief system: that time was of *no essence* (and how could I *not* have thought that, considering our preferred forms of entertainment were those characterized by memory loss and debilitating hangovers). But then the engagements became more frequent. And where it was once a major event to receive a wedding invitation cards were now, on the regular, tainting the rest of my mail (which, when you're thirty, is basically just bills and an *O, The Oprah Magazine*). And then— babies. One by one, my closest confidants gave up their night lives (and, as a result, mine) for night feedings, all for the sake of a homemade nuclear family.

I get it, and I appreciate that all the pregnant women I know are over the moon. It truly is a special and exciting time for everyone, isn't it? The discovery of a new pregnancy can turn even the greatest cynics into temporary optimists as they bask in the fairy-tale version of maternity: radiant skin, the termination of the dreaded calorie count, and the notion of "building a crib with your partner as cartoon birds whistle on the windowsill." But those rose-colored glasses must come from the same faulty line as Cinderella's slippers, because they can only be enjoyed for so long before the harrowing truths of "real life" come into focus: morning sickness, hot flashes, hemorrhoids, unfortunate increases in hair distribution and density (never in the places you would hope), and *sobriety*. Pregnancy can be a buzzkill, and its effects spread far beyond the individual. Believe me, just because there's no offspring throwing up on my clothes, it doesn't mean that my present and future aren't engulfed in babies.

It's clear that my friends, for example the woman who wrote so eloquently in the foreword before mine, are clearly off birth control. Everywhere stomachs are popping, and if you're reading this, yours might be, too. Whether you're ready or not, you are now an active participant in one of the most stressful, hysterical, and fascinating science experiments Mother Nature has to offer. Signing up was the fun part. Moving forward is much trickier. A bun in the oven is a strange and serious business. You'll find yourself saying, doing, and behaving in ways you would have never imagined. Ways that will humor, endear, and hearten those around you, while at the same time alienating, annoying, and antagonizing the hell out of them.

The saving grace is that you choose your own life path, and these choices can be made simpler with a little self-awareness and a lot of hard-truthed guidance. This is where we come in. Your friends might be afraid to tell it "like it is," but among these pages you'll get it straight from the horse's mouth (Allison) and ass (I guess that's me?). I've taken every breath of commentary our duelling "with child" and "without child" perspectives have exchanged over the years and written it *the F* down. All of it. What has emerged is a devilishly sarcastic and emboldened breakdown of each upcoming challenge and milestone, along with the hilarious *do's* and *please, god, don'ts* we feel you must know. So, next time one of your friends claims they could "fill a book" with their policies on maternity and motherhood, tell them it's already been said and done—by us. We really hope you enjoy it.

—*Jillian M. Parsons, a "Non-Mom"*

SECTION 1
THE FIRST TRIMESTER

THE PREGNANCY TEST

Successive Tidal Waves of Emotion
and a Whole New Ballgame

It all begins with a late period. A late period that, like every late period before it, is met with little to no concern. Punctuality is not a period's strong suit. They operate under their own agendas, a large part of which is reserved for being totally unreliable. We women are well versed in the habits of "big red," and it is this know-how that prevents us from losing our goddamn minds whenever our cycles forget to clock in on time. That being said, whether we're keeping a precise tally of period no-shows or not, we always know when we have hit one too many days. *Always.*

Practically every woman has at one time or another believed she was pregnant. Those beliefs result in what we call "mini-scares," which wind down when we receive indication that, once again, we've gotten ahead of ourselves and it's off to the store for another box of Super

Plus tampons (which, by the way, do not represent the size of our vaginas, okay, nosy pervert in the Walmart checkout line). The truth is, children or no children, by the time we hit thirty, *most* of us have shared in the emotionally enormous task of urinating all over the life-changing gadget known as the *EPT*, which stands for *early pregnancy test* (but we will also accept *e-mmidiate panic trigger* as the experience is often accompanied by a raging anxiety attack).

It's hard to keep track of all the benefits of being female, but the nervous energy to which we're referring isn't necessarily a bad thing. The ubiquitous "word on the street" is that there is something called a "planned pregnancy," a phenomenon where women *look forward* to the pee-centric ritual we described earlier. But despite all the joy that can come from urinating on a stick, it's still a pretty unmagical way to discover whether you may or may not be bringing new life into this world—though perhaps it is good practice. A foreshadowing of where you'll be nine months from now (though it's not only "number one" that gets everywhere during childbirth).

The Secret Past of Sexually Active Women

Historically speaking, the EPT is a godsend. A golden shower (on a stick) never hurt anyone, therefore, should your poise waiver during the self-test phase, know that you are one lucky motherf'er. Now, more than ever, is the time to get knocked up.

Before the sexual revolution of the seventies, women weren't allowed to worry within the privacy of their own minds or make decisions about their bodies within the sanctity of their own values. Back then, you had to involve other parties to prove your pregnancy. Parties that were not always other human beings. Parties that were, in some cases, *grain*—as in those small, hard, dry seeds you never once thought about using as a toilet. Our predecessors also dabbled in bulbous and sulfurous vegetables; even rats and rabbits had a role to play in early pregnancy detection. But of course, and much like today, behind the inception of many of these strange practices were misguided males.

This checkered past should be a surprise to absolutely nobody. After reviewing the evidence, it's hard to believe abstinence didn't break out in epidemic proportions that so many women continued perpetuating the human race, given the bizarre hoops they had to jump through and the sheer volume of mansplanations they were forced to concede. Never a dull moment when it comes to the rich history of female subjugation.

Ancient Egypt—The Piss Garden

Have you ever wanted to pee all over a bowl of barley and wheat but always seemed to miss the opportunity? Well, friend, you are living in the wrong millennium because it just so happens that in 1350 BC, anyone who suspected their main man of slipping one past the goalkeeper did just that. If a woman's sprinkle of a tinkle resulted in a sprout, then pregnancy was afoot; but if she couldn't make her garden grow, the poor gal was considered another day barren (*and* incredibly wasteful, considering the needless contamination of community resources). We know, it's so unfair. All we get to fiddle around with is a dopey, plastic wand, while our ancestors were off partaking in light gardening. At least it's relatively inoffensive, right? Would you believe it gets weirder?

Ancient Greece—The "You Want Me to Put *What Where*?" Test

The Greeks know what they are doing when it comes to food; Jillian has always admired their penchant for olives—and those Souvlaki platters are the business. However, a long time ago, in a galaxy no way near far enough away, everyone was getting *completely* carried away with the level of intimacy they afforded their ingredients. For instance, as a precursor to impregnation, the Greek woman was advised to place an onion (or garlic,—

her body, her choice) into her vagina before bedtime to determine her ability to conceive (how cozy!). If she awoke in the morning with the pungent allium on her breath, she was supposedly good to go.

Whoa. Pump the breaks, Greece. This is unfortunate for so many reasons and *so many people.* Our hearts go out to this poor girl—and her partner. Though there's no way to be sure, garlic *probably* doesn't come out of vagina on the first, or even second, wash. And is it just us, or is it beginning to sound like this methodology had a lot less to do with science and a lot more to do with misogyny, for example, the revenge plot of a spurned ex-lover (that got way too out of hand) resulting in a nationwide kibosh on cunnilingus? Because if it is one of those rare instances where a "so crazy it just might work" plan *actually* worked? Well, at least that makes sense, and may we just say: Well played, sir.

The Germans—AKA the Rabbit Killers

The twenties may not seem that far behind us, but what you're about to read will not only cause you to feel the distance between now and then; you'll also feel the distance between here and another planet. Just shy of a century ago, doctors in Germany were going through a shit-ton of mice, rats, and, yes, bunnies in order to oust potential mothers-to-be. The Germans would inject women's urine into any of the three unlucky critters, eventually killing them (the critters, not the women). This was followed by a search for traces of the pregnancy hormone *hCG* via an internal investigation of the ovaries (again, of the critters, not the women).

That would have to amount to a lot of animal testing. Yuck. But it happened, and you can thank this SNAFU for the idiom "the rabbit died," which means that someone is pregnant. Wait, what? That term isn't in the family building vernacular you're familiar with? Because you're not over ninety? Wake up! The roaring twenties wasn't all hobnobbing with Great Gatsbys and smoking from ridiculous cigarette holders that dangled your dart two feet in front of your face; it was also about rubbing shoulders with mad scientists, making it a dark time for our gender and, lest we forget, the local animal population.

How to Wrangle Your Intel 101

Enough with the regressive history lessons. Let's talk about what happens next, when your radar is going off and you are faced with a possible pregnancy, pre-EPT. During these early stages, only your closest friends are made aware of the potentially realized bundle of cells. There are numerous ways in which women choose to pass along this information, but let's make an ass out of you and we and assume you blew up the inner circle with a couple of texts. Something along the lines of "I'm late . . ." or the less cagey version, "I THINK I'M FUCK-ING PREGNANT." Whoever is on the receiving end of those loaded messages is going to have to read between the lines. Fear doesn't mean you can't be equally excited, and vice versa. Friends *will* pay attention to your tone (when speaking) or punctuation (when typing away feverishly on your mobile) in hopes of giving you the most appropriate response, but mistakes can be made and reactions can fall flat, making everything seem worse.

For the woman in question, as long as the support system can project an absurd amount of enthusiasm (not unlike those unhinged adults starring in children's morning shows), everyone should be off to a promising start. If you're feeling elated by the discovery, you'll likely be *juuuust* fine. But if you're having difficulty reaching a state of euphoria (as in it's early evening and you're giving yourself morning sickness just thinking about morning sickness), than some coddling may be in order. Let's examine how both scenarios can play out and how each will undoubtedly result in friends and family unintentionally misstepping all over your moment, regardless of whether you're tickled pink or feeling blue.

"I May Be Pregnant :)"

Check out that smiley face! Someone's having a good day! So, you're pleased with the prospect of being in the family way. That's great. If you've notified the gang via text, we'll assume that you've incorporated emojis to elevate your message, i.e., the baby bottle, a GIF of crying Kim Kardashian, or perhaps something from the Pusheen Eats collection. Nothing says "I'm taking this seriously!" like a trail of nonsensical cartoons at the end of a life-changing announcement. This period of uncertainty is fleeting, so remember to soak it up in the most annoying ways possible. Everyone is "here for you" now more than ever before, and they'll serve as your emotional amplifiers, dancing hand-in-hand with you all the way to the doctor's confirmation. Are you totally pumped? Then they're totally pumped. As long as you can keep it up, they will, too.

"I May Be Pregnant :("

Uh-oh, the frowny-face. This situation can be precarious. Listen, even planned pregnancies have been known to rock the emotional system. If this is you, expect tears, hyperventilation, properly deliberation, and contemplation that can only be done properly while gazing painstakingly out of a window on a rainy day (why you, why him, why now, etc.). Whenever friends receive these outcries, the emojis we mentioned earlier are tabled, and in their place is a grab bag of everyone's favorite expletives. This is not to take away from women who broach their pregnancy with hesitation; on the contrary, it is, and definitely always will be, okay to *not* be okay as reality sets in. Hey, it's a big deal! Biology has essentially sentenced you to a year of non-alcoholic beer and weight gain, and all because you were horny that *one* time. Of course, the worries and sob fests are followed up by what some call the "ultimate reward"—a baby. Yes, that's right, you're going to have a baby! But we digress.

To the Drugstore!

If you're taking the approach of "what I don't acknowledge eventually goes away," we're going to have to stop you right there. This isn't Saturday night, and your pregnancy is not the guy across the bar whose stare feels like he's trying to lobotomize you with his eyes. There's a difference between trying to keep things on the DL to prevent word from spreading and trying to keep things on the DL in hopes of some sort of mysterious "resolution." As much as some people wish that were an option, *it's just not how it works*, and most of us can only commit to that level of delusion for so long before enlisting friends to gather the provisions needed to get to the root of your uterine puzzle.

Playing personal shopper isn't as embarrassing a gig for your friends as you might think. We're all adults now, right? So, what if a minor acquaintance decides to tell the world about someone's not-so-stealthy shopping trip down the sexual health aisle? It's not like they're picking up an oral herpes remedy. Honestly, if this were a game of "Would You Rather?," every woman would go for "caught red-handed with fistfuls of EPTs" over "seen hovering suspiciously by the cold sore medication." And hey, if word does get out, it's the sort of rumor that resolves itself in time. So, since you have your gal pals right where you want them, you might as well put them to work. They will do whatever you want, whatever you need, and whatever it *takes* to get you full of fluids and into a bathroom, armed with the necessary gear to put an end to the guesswork.

Analog or Digital; OMG, It Doesn't Matter

There are different ways of finding out if one is or if one isn't, and you have a few options:

a) How you want to pee; are you partial to peeing *onto* or *into* things?

b) How the results are delivered; are you able to discern between one line and two, or are you an idiot?

Speaking of idiots, we've *both* taken pregnancy tests before, and we *always* go for the high-tech, one-button-away-from-being-a-Texas-Instrument kit. The digital versions just feel more accurate, and sometimes we need things literally spelled out for us in high-stress situations. Regardless of which winds up between your legs, just like choosing where to grab dinner when you're starving, quantity should trump quality. Buy a lot. You should have an unlimited salad bar's worth of pregnancy tests in there with you. They say there is power in numbers, and one positive or negative outcome often isn't deemed reliable enough by those being verified (even though it usually is). It isn't called a test for nothing. You are going to want to check your work. And then recheck it. And maybe recheck it again. (No need to compare results with your friends; it will only add to the confusion.)

You're Pregnant!(?)

Not to add insult to injury, but this is only the beginning, and we mean that in both a threatening and compassionate way. Depending on your readiness, you're either going to be uber- excited, marked by unintelligible scream-crying and other abrasive displays of glee, *or* you will appear to be doing your most uncanny "deer caught in headlights while secretly willing the car to accelerate" impression. In this case, everyone should postpone the jumping up and down and shrieking celebratory words such as "Yay" or "Congratulations." It's too soon and much too severe. Best for family and friends to tread softly and be extra generous with appeasing pats on the back. Presents are also welcome distractions. If any of the multiple shoulders being cried on should have unused gift cards taking up space in their wallets, now would be a good time to play them. Nothing can brighten even the most shocking of days like a little retail therapy.

Friends Won't Pass the Whisper

The intel remains close to the chest for some time, and keeping the big secret is a real hoot for those "in the loop." (FYI, *hoot* means "a good time," and if you're planning on becoming a mom, you're going to have to find a way to work it into your vocabulary.)

Covering up the tracks of your AWOL menstrual cycle is no small potatoes, but it *does* give pals an excuse to bust out their oversized floppy hats and tap into the international-woman-of-mystery tricks one can only acquire by watching countless hours of PBS's *Where in the World is Carmen Sandiego*. And trickery will come into play. Ordering mocktails on the sly is harder than you think, and we should know. We've both been known to sneak a few near-beers into our nights out on the town, and they never, ever go unnoticed, at least not by the hawkeyed jezebels we run with. Unfortunately, you have no choice but to cut out that sweet, sweet alcohol completely—and it won't end there. You will have to abstain from processed meats (bye-bye spamwiches!) and ghost your favorite sushi haunt (which can be explained away by imaginary IBS flare-ups, though less embarrassing excuses work, too).

Whatever you come up with, you can count on friends to do their absolute best to keep the cat sealed tightly inside the bag. Anything to prevent thwarting your big surprise or, god forbid, ruining your release of an unnecessarily gimmicky pregnancy announcement. Which has already crossed your mind, hasn't it? You've been thinking about it forever. You've done mock-ups in your head, considered fonts, and even envisioned the cherub-like baby you haven't yet birthed, splayed across glossy cardstock. For you, it will serve as the treasured symbol of a precious life event. However, it can represent something quite different for others—such as the first sign of the mental transformation you and every woman before you have suffered as a result of pregnancy: complete and total neurological corny-ification.

EXCESSIVE SALIVA, WIND, AND CONSTIPATION—OH MY!

Does Chanel Make HAZMAT Suits?

You probably still resemble yourself in mind, body, and spirit, but underneath it all, somewhere between your boobs and the bottom of your vagina, changes are already underway. Some of these will go unnoticed, but many of them won't, and it's in these transformations where you'll discover the El Dorado of toilet humor you've spent your whole life searching for (or has it only been us?).

When it comes to uncovering the embarrassing side of motherhood (pre- and post-birth), you need to know what to look for (hint: keep your eyes and ears peeled for terms that would make the "old you" uneasy). Some parenting sites show no fear when sharing the "wait, *what* happens to my perineum?" side of things, and those are the ones worth going over with a fine-toothed comb. We encourage a deep dig, because popular culture has done women a grave disservice in the way it blankets modern maternity in rainbows and butterflies, shining the spotlight on the beauty, mystique, and miracle of procreation. Ask any woman on month eight of her pregnancy how miraculous her ingrown "Rat King of pubic hairs" is feeling (on second thought, let it get infected first). Your next year ahead is going to be a lot less enchanting than advertised. As Yoda once said, "Dark times are these . . ." and man, can they ever be.

You know what? Go ahead and blame the big and small screens for these false impressions. They think they're breaking boundaries whenever they show a lead actress vomiting into a trashcan or having an urge to urinate in a happy-go-lucky sort of way. Just so we're all on the same page, morning sickness is not taboo, nor is properly answering nature's call. And if TV thinks puke and piss constitute "edgy" signs that a character is pregnant, the other side effects that have been left in the dark must be truly horrific. And they are. If you ask anyone who has experienced pregnancy, either first- or secondhand, they'll tell you the physical symptoms can rattle even the most generous comfort levels, trip internal TMI alarm systems, and send "regular people" running for the hills.

It's probably best to keep this at the forefront of your mind: Pregnancy isn't really a miraculous event; it's a scientific one, and science can get super gross. The body's reaction to gestation is way raunchier than anything involving a toilet and much less cool than having a huge rack. Please note, when we say *gross*, we are not referring to packing on a few (or more than a few) pounds: women going from one person to two and gaining a little girth along the way? That's not icky, that's just sound math. We're talking about the side of pregnancy that, we believe, may be the true source of the infamous maternal glow. The side that is overheated. The side that is constipated. The side that is mouthfuls of excessive spit and asses polluting the air so earnestly that if Disney were to ever cast a live-action remake of *Fern Gully*, they would be frontrunners for the role of Hexxus. It's the angle that most people shy away from, and subsequently, the angle we most enjoy playing up. Get out the barf bags, you're going to need them.

You Need to Pee Now—and Always

Between the two sexes, frequent declarations of "needing to pee" is *our* thing, which may explain why this subject is shrouded in the world's worst excuse for mystery. Women can be heard anywhere and everywhere sounding off on their desire to urinate before splitting the scene either as a solo or team effort. Why do we do this? Why does it seem like we're always on our way to, or returning from, a piss party? And when did the single-stall bathroom become our clown car equivalent (the number of women seen spilling out of one at any given time is completely implausible). For many of us, we merely enjoy the company, no matter how "totes inapropes" the venue. But preggos, don't have a choice. You actually have to go. Over and over again.

Speaking of going numero uno, Jillian's sister contributed this juicy nugget of information: Pregnant women pee themselves. It's a shame that's *not* the best short story ever written or the uninspired title of a fairly-tame (and probably dated) fetish porn. Instead, it's just a stone-cold fact. If you don't recognize the signs fast enough, you're in trouble; even a sneeze can leave you in a cesspool of your own making. Classic slapstick, mom style.

Thank god we've spent our whole lives desensitizing those close to us to our lavatory habits. Who's going to care or notice if said habits intensify? We always pee together anyway. So, as long as your wing-women are prepared to accommodate more bathroom trips and arm themselves with sanitary napkins in case your bladder forgets to ask for permission before emptying, accidents have a good chance of being avoided. #Blessed.

Hemorrhoids

Something like 50 percent of pregnant women get hemorrhoids. This is a direct insight taken from a close friend, someone who would rather die than have her name printed in this context. Have you ever had a hemorrhoid? Did you know that hemorrhoids are actually just varicose veins? And did you also know that the only thing worse than varicose veins networking across your gams are the ones that are networking across your taint?

Hemorrhoids, or as they're referred to in layman's terms, hemorrhoids (could nobody come up with a code word?!), are painful, but they're not deadly. We won't say who, but one of us has had hemorrhoids (initials J. P.). They aren't active right now, but who knows what state this undisclosed anus will be in by the time we finish this book (or chapter, for that matter). The thing is, kids or no kids, hemorrhoids happen and can serve as a great conversation piece for a girls' night out or catching up with a loved one via a long-distance Skype date. They are the stand-up comedians of private part problems, but that doesn't mean playing host is going to be a chuckle fest. Don't be afraid to ask your friends if they have any under their own belts (literally and figuratively). Let those who have suffered from the same rectal deformities be your pillar of extra-strength Preparation H (and remind you that you are not abnormal). These uninvited guests will go away (and come back), so there really is no need to feel like a monster (which is hard when you're dealing with a fire-breathing asshole). Might we suggest you do what we all do: use hydrocortisone discreetly and find an excuse that will keep your main man or woman far away from the temporarily out-of-order sexy areas. And wipe very, very, gently. You don't want to upset the hemorrhoids; they are a fickle bunch.

Gas

Gas is hilarious when being expelled by women—particularly women who are trying their damnedest *not* to expel said gas. And know that when we say gas, we are referring to both farting *and* burping. Farting and burping refuse to discriminate, *especially* against pregnant women. In fact, it seems that eructation and flatulence may prefer them.

While spending an afternoon deciding between pizza and Thai food, we decided to solve the age-old question of how many times a day the average person "cuts the cheese." That's right, just your everyday "girl talk," and before you close your eyes and try to carry over digits in your head, the answer is fourteen. We shared this discovery with a friend, who then felt inclined to throw his own favorable bit of trivia into the mix: the amount expressed daily by a single individual is often enough to fill a standard-sized basketball. In case you forgot, basketballs aren't small. And that doesn't even account for those of you who are farting for two . . .

During pregnancy, not only does the internal gas tank we all pretend not to have become fuller than normal, it also feels like it's being topped up at an expedited rate. No one (not least a woman) ever thought to themselves, *I wish I could fart and/or burp more.* That is a lot of hot air to distribute evenly and undetected, and you won't be able to pull it off every time. We all have those days when we are more walking nuclear power plant than feminine seductress, but let us remind you: we are all still human, whether we smell and sound like one—or not.

Pro Tip: If there is someone close to you who is fishing for the title of "Bestie of the Year," here's one way you can help them seal the deal: have them invest in a couple of horns and whistles for those moments when you break out into a trademark fumy rage. With noisemakers already at the scene, that friend can instantaneously pull focus away from the audible mess you've generated. It's like the old saying goes: there's nothing like doing a solid, for a bit of gas.

Constipation, and the Opposite

If you're a grown woman, you're probably already familiar with the chastening experience of constipation and its inverse (which is the most diplomatic term we could think of for "diarrhea"). If adulthood has taught us anything, it's that every woman and her fifteen cats suffer from some sort of intestinal dysfunction. In terms of being backed up, here's how you can "push" for the win: an abundance of fiber and fluids. Think industrial-sized containers of Metamucil, administered by the ladle-full— or beans and anything resembling them, i.e., lentils and split peas. This isn't the orphanage in Oliver Twist; there is no shortage, so get this stuff into you if you want *other* stuff out of you. For the other affliction, the one that starts with a screaming "D," nothing can beat Imodium (or, as Jillian likes to refer to it whenever she frantically ingests multiple doses in a public place: "my goddamn birth control pills—okay?").

Pro Tip: You're going to want to keep the latter in a decoy container. An empty travel-size Q-Tip box usually does the trick. The more paranoid may want to hot-potato it, tacking several layers of paper towel or toilet paper onto the original packaging. Sure, it sounds over-the-top, but many women would do just about anything to avoid that moment when an Imodium Dissolvable tablet falls from our wallet onto a table, exposing our most carefully kept bowel secret.

Your Skin ~~Glows~~ Blows

Everyone has heard that pregnancy skin is *the* skin to have. Remember the "glow" we mentioned earlier? That's real life. We mean it. Moms-to-be truly can beam; it almost hurts the eyes. But don't put all your remaining eggs into the flawless complexion basket (ah yes, *that* old Chinese proverb). Your physiology is about as coherent as a mid-aughts Lindsay Lohan at half-past shots o'clock, so not every pregnancy will give "great face." Or body. The skin is one behemoth of an organ. With all the positive manifestations come negative ones, and whatever abnormalities do arise, expect them almost anywhere and everywhere.

Acne

Acne sucks, but at some point, the pubescent pizza face you thought was well behind you, the one you keep buried in that secret box of high school photographs you have yet to burn, might reemerge. In other words, #FreshFaceFridays could be on the back-burner for a while. This will be difficult for those who were fortunate enough to shake breakouts as they entered their twenties, but some of us weren't so lucky. Many of us *still* suffer through days where we look as if we're doing really poorly in that nineties board game Girl Talk (we *wish* those were stickers), and that's when you turn to your holy grail Benzoyl Peroxide supply and the wonder that is Nars concealer. If you need help in this area, YouTube is bursting with tutorials on how to paint a more familiar visage over the stranger you see in the mirror. But beware: it's not a long trip between good makeup artistry and overdoing it and though no one can predict future trends, we're pretty confident clown-face isn't making it's way down the pipe. So, get to know your way around a makeup brush and be honest about your abilities. If you're thinking you might have gone a little overboard, put down the contour kit and listen to your eyeballs. They don't lie.

Skin Tags

They're like the three-dimensional, abjectly less cute cousin of the freckle; the latter being expressed by sun exposure, and the former being expressed by neglecting to incorporate a condom into bedroom antics. Why

couldn't the people tasked with naming dermatologi-
cal defects decide on something, *anything*, other than
"skin tag"? And what's perhaps even more exasperating
is that the chances of playing host to a plethora of these
things don't only exist; they're high. Just another one of
nature's countless gifts as you embark on your maternal
adventure (and when the adventure ends, you can have
these same gifts removed quickly and easily by a doctor,
thank god).

Hyperpigmentation

The linea nigra, also known as the "pregnancy line," is
a hyper-pigmented streak that extends from belly button to crotch and can be seen on the majority of women
in their final trimester. Friends have characterized it as
"brown and dirty-looking," verbatim, and however vague
that may read (because, let's be honest, it's not the only
thing on the human body fitting the description), it's
pretty damn accurate. For those interested in mixing up
the look of their nether regions but are not yet ready
for the flashiness of vajazzling*, a "brown and dirty-
looking" line could be a good place to start. At least from
there, there would be nowhere to go but up.

------

*Vajazzling: the bedazzlement of the vagina, worn by every nine-
ties boy's wet dream, Jennifer Love Hewitt.*

Stretch Marks

They happen. If you don't get stretch marks during your pregnancy, keep an eye out for them afterwards because once the milk comes in, they usually follow suit. All good things come with a price, and although your big boobs might look *"Sports Illustrated Swimsuit Issue"* worthy when clothed, what lies beneath would be better suited for *The Magazine of Fantasy & Science Fiction* (or science non-fiction in your case, which is just "science"). As Dwight Schrute from *The Office* would say, "Tit for tit." And as Jim Halpert would reply, "That's not the expression."

Hot Flashes

Hot flashes are a damn nuisance. Nothing is worse than being extremely overheated. You never know when or where they'll occur or to what severity, like those sexy pop-up ads paired with suggestive audio that continue to plague your laptop ever since you visited PornHub that *one* time(s).

To sidestep these thermal traps, you need only one thing: common sense. Do what the pre-pregnant you would do whenever she used to get hot: wear natural fibers; take a cool shower; drink some water; and consider investing in one of those spritz-bottle mini-fans. Luckily, you can find both of these at junior soccer tournaments (which, if you're in the city, means every two blocks). So whenever your skin is melting to the ground and you feel like the Wicked Witch of the West, get yourself to the nearest children's sporting event and buy the refreshment stand out from under the young folks. Problem solved(-ish).

Hair

Hair, hair, everywhere. Remember when Liz Lemon revealed her *friend* "Tom Selleck" on *30 Rock*? A friend who turned out to be her naturally occurring mustache that would crop up unless she paid it fastidious attention? Well, this pregnancy has put you at risk . . . of going rogue in the facial hair department and coming face-to-face with your very own "Tom Selleck." Not to mention the nipple hair department, the back of the thighs department, the chin hair department, etc.

These areas require heavy surveillance. Consider starting a discussion among friends (the franker, the better) regarding the level of intervention you expect. Sure, the embarrassment that comes with being told you're only a couple strands away from being nicknamed "Whiskers" can sting, but what would you rather: a mammoth-sized hair being picked up by a friends radar or having to answer a stranger's observational notes with: "No, sorry, that's attached." Accept that memo, as swiftly and privately as possible.

This neighborhood watch will cover most of your follicle-related bases, but there are some areas that are off limits even to our closest confidants. A *really* annoying milestone in your pregnancy will be when your belly grows so big that you have to get a sense of the state of your bush using Helen Keller–like skill. We can think of worse things than saying so long to the visual of your pubic hair (for instance, the visual of your pubic hair); however, "out of sight" should not equate to "out of mind." A woman known to both of us debated asking her husband if he'd custom tailor her meat curtains. Part of her motivation was her inability to style "herself" herself, but mostly she wanted to save doctors from spending the first half of the delivery weed-whacking while her baby was left in the lurch. Bottom line, *somebody* is going to have to think about the bush—but leave chemicals off the table. You don't want your sickeningly sweet-smelling baby's head to come out reeking of *Nair*.

Boobs

Colossal boobs: For all the cons, there is one unanimous pro that comes with pregnancy, and that is "sick" (clap emoji) "cans" (clap emoji). Sure, there may be some stretch marks, and your nipples might take up more residential space than you're used to, but big boobs are super neat (ask any man's last Google search). They're the un-shittiest end of the pregnancy stick, and when your alien form has you down in the dumps, you can buck yourself up by taking stock of the two gargantuan bonuses oozing out of your XXL over-the-shoulder-boulder-holder. You are blousy as hell, and with great bra size comes great enviableness. That porny chest will leave some pals riddled with jealousy, so, here are some things to feel insecure about before you get too comfortable out-boobing your BFFs like a boss:

- Areolas darken, become more noticeably bumpy, and hairier. Yup.
- Because they are about to explode, your boobs become super veiny. They'll look and feel like they're on the brink of self-awareness as they extend their vascular networks in an attempt to take over your entire body and, eventually, the world. The power commanded by pairs like these will make a girl sleep with one eye open, a stark difference compared to the common and much more unexceptional chests that put everybody to sleep (for example, Jillian's).
- With sudden inflation comes the just as sudden deflation, otherwise known as *droopy flapjack syndrome* or *DFS*. But instead of wasting time strolling down "mammary" lane and missing

the big old days, you should be thanking god for push-up bras. They're like extensions for your boobs that add a little more volume during the day while at the same time keeping your nipples contained in a familiar area of your body, i.e., above the belly button.

It's Only Nine Months (Kind of)

Maybe maternity leave isn't only for taking care of kiddos and finding footing among new family dynamics. Maybe it's also a way for moms to hide away from civilization while her body and all its individual parts get back to *her* normal. This is a lot of metamorphosis for one woman, and it might take a little time for the "you" you're searching for to resurface (if you want to return to her at all). We encourage you to stay calm, be patient, and keep your chin(s) up. You can, and will, do this.

A ROSE BY ANY OTHER NAME . . . WOULD BE A ROTTEN NAME FOR A ROSE

You Like What You Like; People Hate What They Hate

Every (honest) woman knows that the real reason most of us want kids (and the only reason those of us who *don't* want kids *want kids*) is because we are holding on to that one great name, a name that demands a legacy—but refuses to work for a cat

At this point, about eight to thirteen weeks in, your little one possesses the proportions of a regulation-sized dust bunny, but it's never too early to kick-start the naming process. It's one of the best parts of being pregnant, primarily because it involves making lists (and making lists is the closest motherhood has come to a crack cocaine equivalent). For once, your irresponsible sexual tendencies are working in everyone's favor as you and your friends relish in the chance to name a teeny-weeny baby!

But before you dive in, check yourself before you wreck ~~yourself~~ your *child's* life. You are *not* in your natural headspace. While your body focuses on making a new brain (from scratch), you are barely getting proper use out of the original copy. Your reason and rationale have been masked by a thick bank of the "baby foggies," and only bits and pieces are getting through. As a precautionary measure, why not informally appoint a few of your gals as "name regulators"? Specifically, the ones who remain proprietors of vacant uteri and are thereby immune to the early onset of "Mom brain." They will do their absolute best to keep you from taking any hard rights or lefts to crazy town, while disguising their dismissals and personal preferences as "helpful" or "in the best interests of the child"—if you throw out life-shattering names like *Coriander* or *Moon-Unit*.

Axing All Things Sarah, David, and E-(Double Consonant)-A

Some names are terrible, and in the baby naming world, "popular" and "terrible" are interchangeable adjectives. Does anyone even know a Sarah anymore? No. You know a Sarah A., Sarah B., and Sarah C. through Z. In the words of South Park Elementary's Annual Comedy

Awards Show host Jimmy Valmer: *"Come. On."* Has everyone forgotten *Sarah, Plain and Tall*? How, out of the zillion other choices, are so many of us still coming back to the oh-so-overdone? And it's not just "Sarahs" who are played out—there's a whole slew of overused first names spread across the last few decades. To be frank, the insertion of an initial is not an acceptable way of creating differentiation in a child's name. Nobody likes the person with the tagalong letter. It's agitating, and it brings us to public enemy number one: cut out every name appearing in any top ten list compiled within your lifetime. That means leaving all links resembling the below examples unclicked:

"Top 10 Cutest ..."
"Top Ten Celebrity ..."
"Hipster Parents' Guide to ..."
"Most Popular Names of ..."

These are what we call red flags, and so should you. Trendiness is the opposite of timelessness. Do not pander to the fads—they come with a shelf-life. These days, being too current can bring you all the way back around to cliché. Instead, listen to your friends. They will hold you back by the collar while you grab at huge mistakes. So, no Ella or Emma. Nix Jacob and Jasper. Next.

Boys and Girls and Birls and Goys

The great thing about "the noughties" is that the name game is undergoing some serious Jedi-mind-trick-like gender bending. There really aren't any "strictly boy" or "strictly girl" names anymore. In this age of gender fluidity, your possibilities are greatly expanded, and the progressiveness doesn't end there. With a few letter swaps, you can turn a stale boy's name into a serious power move for your little girl-to-be (or vice versa). For example:

Traditional Boy's/Contemporary Girl's
Adrian/Adrienne
Charlie/Charlee or Charleigh
Harlan/Harlynne
James/Jaymes
Danny/Dani
Elliot/Elliotte
Payton/Peyton

How easy is that? That's the beauty of modern society; you have the permission to massacre hundreds of perfectly agreeable names in your quest for pseudo-originality (and very real pretension). For instance, we once spent a summer nanny-ing for a wealthy family whose daughter was named Stuart—true story. Stuart evokes about as much femininity as one of those Old Spice gift sets you pick up for Dad as a last resort, "I forgot" Father's Day present—but in this poor woman's case, it worked. It worked because it had to. The birth certificate was signed, sealed, and delivered, and any chance of reconsideration was long behind him, we mean, *her*. Semantics.

Dare to Be Different

It pays to steer away from anything too out-there, but at the same time there's nothing wrong with giving yourself a moment to cultivate your quirky side. Not only can this be amusing for others, but sometimes the truest gems are only stumbled upon when you go way, way outside the box. When considering something odd, or something that sounds like it emerged along with you from the rabbit hole of your last chemical high, lean in. Some friends may even egg you on (for their own entertainment purposes).

If you're anything like us, you already have a stash of never-before-said-together syllables (a stash started long before you became sexually active, much less pregnant). And the inclination to toy with familiar words by taking them miles outside of their socially accepted context only strengthens with age. For instance, Jillian's sister and her carrot-topped husband briefly attached themselves to the name *Pumpkin* "for a little girl" (as if *that* makes it right). Not sure what that would be "for short," but it was definitely *Pumpkin* "for long." It's a doozie, alright, but if she had presented it alongside, say, a painfully generic *Savannah* or *Taylor*, Jillian may have warmed to it. As it turns out, *Pumpkin* has been scrapped and there will never be a Pumpkin Parsons. You know when people say: "It's probably for the best"? Sayings like that were made for situations like this.

You don't have to re-invent the wheel. If slicing up the alphabet or paying homage to popular holiday gourds isn't your cup of tea, you can always take common names and make them better (or, in some instances, worse). Take the evolution of *Maxine* into *Makseen*, whose existence we have validated by a reliable source (Jillian's college roommate). Sure, it's not the most beautiful glow-up, or even a mildly attractive one, but it demonstrates perfectly how, with a few subtle tweaks, any name can be taken from day to night.

But maybe you already have a style that works for you. If you consider yourself a country woman, then you are likely hell-bent on A) having a little girl, B) having said little girl's name end with "i" and C) following that *i*-ending name with the caboose of all redneck names:

"-Lynne." Nothing classes up a *Brandi* or a *Rikki* like a "dash *Lynne*." Friends should be grateful to wash their hands of this one, because man is this mom going to feel that heat when her child (inevitably) files for emancipation on grounds of "reckless identity assignment."

Or maybe you're someone who places yourself above the rest of us and likes to assert your superiority with name suggestions like *Belvedere* or *Montgomery*. These Mamas often adopt the "celebrity approach," which is a shame because when you scrutinize the choices of the rich and famous, it's clear they're flying blind with the rest of us. Gwyneth Paltrow named her baby after a fruit (Apple. *Apple*. Maybe she likes apples, maybe it's the only thing she eats in a day, unless it's not organic, in which case she'll just have the bowl of free-range steam). Alec Baldwin and Kim Basinger named their daughter after a whole country (Ireland). Kate Hudson named her youngest son after absolute nonsense (Bing). Other stars seem drawn to colors (Beyoncé and Jay Z's *Blue* or Jennifer Garner and Ben Affleck's *Violet*).

It all boils down to one hell of a spectrum of possibilities, but our point remains: you have the potential to do serious damage to your innocent offspring, even before they're born. Irreversible damage or, at least, irreversible apart from legal intervention. For god's sake, try to stay semi-grounded.

Different . . . But Not Too Different

Different is good. But too different is sometimes not. Let's start with the latest and greatest in first name decor: apostrophes. Avoid any name that has more than a couple of these squirrely little bastards. O'Conner? Okay. De'W'Ayne? Maybe. But D'K'Ota? While we're at it, why not see if you can incorporate all fourteen of American English's punctuation symbols. To be fair, names like these can and do work, when it is culturally appropriate. Otherwise, they come off as fussy and disorienting.

Speaking of points of cultural difference, Allison's husband is Dutch, and we're not sure if you're aware, but the Dutch language is *quite* different from the one you're currently reading. That's a fact (and also an excuse Allison's Dutch teacher is *really* sick of hearing). When it came time to name their daughter, even though he pushed for ones representative of his homeland, the risk of chronic-mispronunciations was too great. Can you say *Lieneke* out loud and confidently at the same time? Neither can we, though it was his top contender. Ultimately, Allison and her husband went with Vera—classic, sweet, and only four simple letters. Vera is what you would call a low-risk name, and if someone struggles with it, well, that struggle probably wasn't their first of their day.

Silent letters that sneak into what would otherwise be an easy-to-say-and-spell name can also be trouble.

Isla (pronounced "eye-la") may appear distinctive, but know that you are setting your kid up for a lifetime of corrections. Even if you couldn't care less (it's not your problem, right?), don't be tempted to let it lie. Though we suppose things could and have been worse, case in point: the very real-life sob story of Hashtag, a bouncing baby boy born in the UK whose name, while not containing any silent letters, gives voice to the pound sign. That's right, first name "Hashtag," last name "Wait . . . what?" The real question is how, out of the seven billion or more people on the planet, did the only two people willing to name their child Hashtag find each other? Anything would be better; literally, the word *anything* would be a better name for a human baby than *Hashtag* Dang.

Middle Name Rodeo

The middle name is truly the Bermuda triangle of the full name, from which only the mononymous are safe. Whatever gets slipped into this space is often never heard of again. Even with age, the haunting continues. We all know one, two, or many otherwise mature adults who refuse, under every circumstance, to give up the goods. This is because a second-rate middle name is a burden you cannot outgrow and is frequently a direct consequence of another one of life's inescapable burdens: family.

For reasons nobody cares about anymore, the middle name is where many parents feel pressure to pay tribute to their ancestry. That's fine; but there's a big difference between honoring and playing fast and loose with tradition. Your son doesn't need three middle names so your father, grandfather, and father-in-law are evenly represented. Dad, Pops, and the other guy are just going to have to get over themselves, so you can spare your child the injustice of a cacophonous mishmash of old-man names. Your best bet? Say the first, middle, and last names out loud, and together. If it doesn't flow, let the middle name(s) go. They are never missed.

Now the Kids Won't Laugh

Another reason to say the whole name aloud is the dreaded nickname. Baby brain might make you miss the obvious. Friends should be on the lookout for bad combos and potential ruin. You can't name your son Mike if your last name is Hunt. If your surname is Little, Richard may be out; no one is going to give Little, Dick a break when they see him on the grad list (nor should they). And while we're at it, avoid incriminating initials. Bailey Jean may seem cute and timely, but anyone with the initials BJ can tell you that, with little forethought, a lot of teasing later in life could have been avoided. Really, any name that warrants its own censor bar shouldn't make it past the preliminary rounds. (Mike Hunt is a fantastic name, though.)

And If Everyone Hates the Name

If you've considered all of the above and still settle on something no one approves of, remember this: when the judge decides, the case is closed. This is going to be your kid's name for his or her entire life, and it's your maternal right to exercise carte blanche. Have fun, don't panic, and go with those guts we're always either listening to or complaining about. Because, really, what do the rest of us know anyway?

THE ULTRASOUND

Or Your (Inevitable) Hysterectomy's "Before" Shot

It may seem like the book is leaning this way, but we *swear* the first three months of pregnancy are not just one huge fart. Many people claim that there are other more sentimental things worth exploring. Have you ever thought to yourself, after watching a tear-jerking romance or seeing a couple in love out in public, *I want to be someone's everything?* Well, get pregnant. You immediately become someone's food, water, shelter, and even their toilet (so scratch that off the bucket list). Women become their baby's world. And what kind of world would that be, you ask? Look no further than the ultrasound.

Is it just us or does it feel as if with every passing year our "womb areas" rouse less and less excitement among others? Likely because newer and fresher uterine real estate has entered the marketplace and taken over ours, what we consider the "old stomping grounds."

And although some of you have been lucky enough to hit the genetic lottery and are still a sizzling commodity, it is our experience that the appeal of our uteri has been on a downswing for some time. Now, you may think this is an irreversible trajectory (apart from using one of those "rejuvenation" procedures or a time machine), but the good news is—it's not. If you throw a baby into the equation, your internal love nest springs right back onto everyone's radar! That's one way to create a buzz, right? And the excitement will follow you everywhere you go, even to the radiology unit!

The first of these visits is generally scheduled before the twentieth week, and if you've never had to get an ultrasound before, it may be your first true glimpse at your inner workings (apart from trying to see down your throat or any other orifice that's piqued your perverted curiosity over the years). This event is often described as *momentous*, but frankly, seeing a completely articulated human form inside one's own can be, in a word, jarring (maybe it's because some of us never aspired to become our very own set of Russian dolls). Whatever it is, we're sure your experience will ultimately leave you love-struck, and not emotionally scarred by the image of a "Nesting Woman" plucked from the pages of the worst Stephen King novel never to be made.

How Many Is a Crowd?

When it comes to ultrasound appointments, anyone and everyone goes, whether it's your partner, your #BFF4Life, or your probation officer. Whether a public or private practice, the maternity community understands the comfort of a "plus-one." Hey, maybe the holier-than-thou "institution of marriage" should take note, specifically those jackass friends who make anyone who happens to be "in-between soulmates" attend their twelve-hour weddings *alone*. At least the ultrasound industry is starting out on the right foot.

You should prepare your tagalongs for a very "revealing" ride. That's the best word to describe it. This is when you learn how much time you have before your little kidney bean's vaginal escape, as well as how many beans (if more than one) will be making their getaway. We hope you're well-versed in sharing, because family members come out of the woodwork when there are whispers of burgeoning offspring, with the more obtrusive ones lurking about like hyenas throughout the entire prenatal period, begging for the inside scraps scoop. They want to know as much as possible: "How's the gestational sac? Amniotic fluid looking good?" Real questions that are *really* nobody else's business—not the local fuel attendant or the pre-pubescent crossing guard—but yours.

Email My ~~Heart~~ Uterus

Modern technology . . . what a trip, eh? Loved ones can no longer complain about issues of distance or "missing out." The tele-ultrasound allows mothers to dial as many as *ten* households directly into their swimsuit areas, which is as crazy as it is impressive. Here's a question: just because you *can* distribute a video link that allows loved ones to follow your sonogram in real-time, does that mean you *should*? We understand the desire to push prints; that's old school. Admitting group tours into one's nether regions, though, seems like a bone that need not be thrown. But you're going to lob it out there anyway, aren't you?

2-D, 3-D, 4-D, Blue Fish

The images of various wombs generated by run-of-the-mill ultrasounds are completely interchangeable. We know it's true, your friends know it's true, and now you do, too. For example; let's say a group of pregnant women tossed all their sonograms into a hat, shook that hat around, and were asked to retrieve their contribution. It wouldn't be easy. Those women would be left gawking at little 8x10s with such earnest perplexity, you'd swear they were holding miniature Magic Eye 3-D illusion cards. Not that you shouldn't bother to print your gritty, low-res fridge ornament, or be proud of what it represents. These tiny talismans carry a supreme amount of significance, but they don't really "paint" anyone "a picture." To do that, one would have to, quite literally, *paint a picture*, which sounds to us like a great way to set baby's first picture apart from all those other oh-so-predictable ultrasound photos. And really, if every pregnant woman tapped into her inner Picasso, prenatal portraits might have a fighting chance of becoming just as arresting to outsiders as they are to insiders! Don't you love pipe-dreaming?

Realistically, though, the two-dimensional, Rorschach-looking versions aren't going anywhere anytime soon, but more and more options are arising. There are add-ons, up-sells, and private practices cropping up around every corner. The most notable advance, which can be seen all over Facebook feeds, is the 3-D snap, which provides an extremely lifelike view of your little one. We all remember the dancing baby from *Ally McBeal*, right? The one who pranced around to the *ooga-chaka, ooga-ooga ooga-chaka* part of "Hooked on a Feeling"? Well, that's kind of like what these high-tech systems generate. And just like its predecessor, everyone is already very tired of them.

We really need to hand it to the tech wizards, though, for throwing down buzzwords like "anatomical realism," which, by the way, is *not* a creative movement driven by nineteenth-century Europeans but rather how they describe lifelike previews of your baby's bod. Now you can see if your little one has your nose, your eyes, maybe even your lips, at least that's what the advertisements say. What you'll *really* be able to see is if your baby *has* a nose, two eyes, or a pair of lips. Trying to pin down a family resemblance at the age of minus-one is reaching, to say the least, and we advise you to approach with caution. This can be where the first seeds of helicopter parenting are sewn, where children fall under high-def observation by Moms even before birth. Remember: even the unborn need space from time to time. Practice restraint, now; you're going to need it later.

On top of all of this sci-fi paraphernalia, you can also sign yourself up for a 3-D video of your baby, an MPEG-4 you'll likely watch on a loop for the next few months or so but that everyone else is only willing to see once. Please don't take a person's limited interest to heart. When friends turn your indie-flick away after the fifth (or fifteenth) time you've pushed it on them, it's not because they have something against your baby, it's because they're starting to develop "something" against you. Don't be shocked when, if you keep it up, said friends come sidling up to you with a video of their own, maybe a recording of their cat waiting by a window or ten on-the-edge-of-your-seat minutes of their niece's hamster struggling to get out from under its water bottle. Think twice the next time you reach for your iPad; your audience might be just as armed (and boring), too.

Finding Out the Sex

An ultrasound can take the guesswork out of whether it's going to be a Chris or Christina, if that's what you're after. If you decide to wait, know that everyone around you is about to magically acquire their own certificate in diagnostic medicine, blindsiding you with completely incognizant gender predictions based on old wives' tales. You will humor these members of your family and friends by allowing them to wave wedding bands over your belly or standing at attention while they examine your pupils for dilation (dilated means "boy" or, more accurately, nothing.)

If you're not cool with strangers telling you it's a chick because you're carrying high, you better find out the sex yourself. Note that ultrasound technicians have been wrong in the past (a three-millimeter penis can be easy to miss), which can lead to delivery room drama on the big day. Some people have even sued after a botched sex prediction—not because it's the smart thing to do, but because they are embarrassments to themselves and society. Rule of thumb: do not be the new mom who takes overworked and undervalued hospital staff to court. Be happy, not petty.

Put Away All the Bad Jokes

If you plan on staying in your sonographer's good book, there are some things you need to avoid saying when kicking back in their chair. You may feel your pregnancy is one of a kind, but this isn't your technician's first rodeo. It's more like his or her twelfth rodeo, of the day, and the last thing they want to do is entertain a smart ass. Inane questions and comments such as, "Will it still be black and white after it's born?" or "Oh, *that's* the umbilical cord?!" aren't going to land well. The imaging wing is not a Laugh Factory. Besides, the person peering into your belly has heard it all before, and if that isn't enough to stop you, consider this: jokes about well-endowed babies are weird, especially when the baby is your own.

DIY Ultrasound

Jillian has been saying for years that somebody needs to develop an at-home Pap smear. Its invention would benefit the many women who for a lifetime have avoided these appointments out of fear and at risk of their well-being. But there is no "Be Your Own Gynecologist" kit (unless you count every household's salad tongs and jar of Q-tips). They have, however, developed one for "Be Your Own Sonographer."

Bringing a portable ultrasound device into the home means you can listen for baby's beating heart any hour of the day and whichever day of the week, granting Moms the ability to surveil their womb twenty-four-seven. But since not all of us are doctors, those without a license should be discouraged from taking this route. Professionals aren't just there for show (although there are times when it would seem that way); they're there so you have someone to blame if things go wrong. Don't miss out on the opportunity to pass the buck of your baby's well-being. Leaving the important details in someone else's more qualified hands will bring you peace of mind, because nothing is more relaxing than the ability to hold others accountable instead of yourself.

And You've Made It

Coming off your first ultrasound often means you are coming out of your first trimester. With a bit of luck you are still unscathed, and with a lot of luck you are still optimistic. The next stage is when the physical and emotional shifts really take hold and where hiding your pregnancy can go on no longer. The second trimester is when you will have to face you and your baby's future head on, equipped with your very own grainy image—a token of hope to clutch along the way. And you better hold on tight; you ain't in Kansas anymore.

SECTION 2
THE SECOND TRIMESTER

DECLARING YOUR MATERNITY (AND SOMEONE ELSE'S GENDER)

A Pregnancy Announcement
as Endearing as a Hangnail

With an ultrasound making the rounds, pregnancy announcements are sure to follow. And let us just say, *wow*. These things have really "taken off." With the Internet enabling everyone to cast their social nets wider than ever, mothers have changed not only how they distribute the details of a new pregnancy, but also to whom (or should we say, to how many). More often than not, a declaration of maternity over social media turns something that was once a charming and relatively closed celebration into a whole new animal. An animal that doesn't feel celebratory at all. An animal that is at times irritating and that stirs up emotions similar to those experienced when somebody coughs or sneezes in your face without warning *or* covering their mouths.

Blame the Internet and handheld devices. Now everything anyone ever does however trivial, is worthy of a freaking broadcast. Had an egg for breakfast? Post it on Instagram. Caught a whiff of an absolutely unwelcome scent on the bus today? Tweet that shit. Fifty-nine hours and nine minutes away until your BFF's return from spending a "nobody cares" amount of time abroad? Status update y'all! We showboat the monotony of daily life as if it is made up of consistently noteworthy events. And we do this everyday, which means that when we *do* find ourselves amid a truly momentous occasion (i.e., expecting a child), we publicize it as if it were part of that same monotony.

For example, following a week's worth of statuses beginning with "That moment when you [insert predictable text]," by the time you finally post an announcement of "We're pregnant!" emblazoned across a clichéd shot of a tiny sneakers, it's already too much and even Celine Dion would roll her eyes.

There has got to be a better way. There *used* to be a better way!

The Pregnancy Announcement: In Simpler Times

Ask your parents how much time, thought, and energy they put into informing their family, friends, acquaintances, the neighbors, and everyone else who ever crossed their path that they were with child. Really—do it. We're guessing they'll say somewhere between none and *maybe* twelve minutes of glib discussion. Back then, finding out that a woman was expecting was just as thrilling, and the mechanics of pregnancy remained the same, but it was a more personal and private affair. Public displays of pregnancy only occurred after someone's belly popped, which was all that was required to alert the masses. People aren't stupid; their eyes tell them all they need to know. Seriously, have you ever seen someone who was obviously pregnant and been unsure if they were obviously pregnant? Not really—except in the rare moment you give up your seat to a "pregnant" woman on the train, only to offend an innocent bystander who just happens to have a bit of girth.

Pregnancy announcements used to be communicated via phone calls (we're talking rotary style) or by verbal exchange, also known as talking to one another, face-to-face. The flashier couples would *maybe* take out an ad in a local paper for the sake of some short-lived notoriety. Once women were able to get over the intimidation that comes with notifying her and her partner's parents, the rest unfolded in a very sincere and organic way. Imagine informing someone of a pregnancy in a deliberately personalized manner. When was the last time that was achieved or, hell, even attempted?

The Pregnancy Announcement: Today

There are those (moms) who insist that modern-day pregnancy announcements are more inclusive, eventful, and fun. You know what? You get two out of the three. Inclusive? Someone has a gift for understatement. Eventful? So eventful it's killing us. But *fun*? That depends on so, so much.

Special information deserves a special delivery, as well as a special audience. Blasting a photo update to the widespread scope of your social network, be it Facebook or Instagram, feels the *opposite* of special. Words like *tacky* and *trite* come to mind. You might not want to believe it, but most users are now completely desensitized by the onslaught and scroll through pregnancy announcements with the same speed (if not more) used to whip past Grumpy Cat memes and the ERMEGHERED girl. It might be a shame, but you have to admit, mother or not, few can care about that many pregnancies.

To be clear, we both enjoy receiving alerts from loved ones who are happy and hopeful about starting their families. Like when Jillian's sister sent her ultrasound through text as they sat together at the kitchen table. Even though Jillian deleted it immediately because the image *appeared* to be broken, her sister sent it again and forced her to pay it some damn attention. Then, in true Parsons' fashion, they both cried. It's absolutely an honor to be a part of big news. That being said, allow us to preface the following paragraphs by saying that as many ways as there are to go about pregnancy updates, the less-than-ideal ways are always the fastest, easiest, and unfortunately the most common.

The Gender Reveal

It's the latest fad, it's all the rage, it's the "Gender Reveal"! This is no longer something that is simply "said." Gone are the days of disclosing the sex in the banality of everyday conversation. Now, friends get to sit back and wait for you to *show* them! It's also an excuse to get friends together again, especially since your girls' nights out and hangover brunches have come to a standstill ever since the pregnancy announcement kicked alcohol out of the equation (you take booze out of any relationship and things are going to *slow down*). Plus, the baby shower just seems *too* far away, and you need to squeeze another party in. It's not like anyone will have the nerve to turn you down. Pregnant women have everybody right where they want them—they have them by their guilt.

To be fair, not every mom will draw out the gender reveal, but *lots* do. If you decide to go all out, you'll likely kick things off with a countdown, keeping everyone on their toes. As a favor to friends, don't start with too far away from the date, for example, two weeks out. Frankly, that's exhausting, and by the time fourteen days come and go, the whole mystique will have played itself out. Plus, let's be honest, there is limited mystique to begin with. We're dealing with only two possible outcomes. Three days is a much safer allotment of time.

Following the countdown conclusion, a stunt is often put in place to unveil the results. Maybe a cord will be pulled and blue or pink balloons will fall from your ceiling. Maybe you and your partner will have fists full of appropriately colored confetti you plan to blow into the faces of your unsuspecting (and pretty soon unimpressed) guests. Or maybe you will rent a projector from the local junior high and flash either a penis or a vagina onto your living room wall, making yours the most X-rated gender reveal of all time. Either way, we predict theatrics. It sounds over-the-top, but the payoff for guests will be the ample finger foods and refreshments you *better* provide. Because if people can't count on the pregnant lady for a proper feed, who can they count on?

If We Can't Beat 'Em, Bail

The most common reaction we see to post-millennial pregnancy and gender announcements are more jeers than cheers. It's the heavy-handed exorbitance being demonstrated; it's *too* much. We're not saying anyone needs to be muzzled, but there is all sorts of middle ground between being a boisterous blowhard and taking an oath of silence. The best way to avoid behind-the-back disapproval of your peers is to be a traditionalist (which actually makes you ahead of your time). Find a method that is both fun and authentic, or whatever word is the antonym to a face palm. Don't be afraid to turn to gal pals when you're looking for a voice of reason—that way, when it's all said and done, everyone will be impressed by your knack at keeping things simple.

BABY BRAIN

You No Think Good No More

When this new side of your personality emerges, there will be no mistaking it. The changes will be subtle in the beginning, going unnoticed under the guise of everyday mishaps—maybe you totally butcher the name of your favorite pop star or completely space out on a Tuesday coffee date thinking it's Thursday. Shit that could happen to anyone. But then one day you leave a voicemail on a friend's machine that was clearly meant for your mother, and you pop into your doctor's appointment with your pants wide open, unbuttoned, and unzipped (here's hoping you remembered the underwear). When you start adding all these incidents together, you're left with the diagnosis staring you right in the face. It's chronic, degenerative, and incurable. It's early-onset Mom Brain, aka Baby Brain.

Baby Brain is when your mind slowly turns to mush as you house a baby in your belly. Your cognitively adept self recedes, and a new brain, version 2.0, takes over. Actually, let's knock that 2.0 down to a 0.5. The greater number implies an upgrade, and that's not a word we would use to describe the situation. It's a mental demobilization, eventually leaving you with only goopy, indecipherable to-do's and reflections as your dicey brainwaves merge into one homogenized pool of indistinguishable thought.

It sounds scary, but because it's as common as it is damaging, you will never be alone in the fight. Every mom suffers from this from one degree to another, and it has caused some pretty ridiculous stories to circulate. Luckily, these moments can be blamed on your unborn baby. (Post-birth is all about blaming the baby for *not* being able to do shit; pre-birth is about blaming the baby for *doing* stupid shit.) Unluckily, having an excuse doesn't always make things easier. Becoming forgetful and disorganized can be hard for those who are used to regimented living. Losing track of plans, objects, people, and time is frustrating and dispiriting, and it takes maximum efforts to conceal it. As the due date nears, your train(s) of thought are likely to go off the rails. Your partners-in-conversation will become lost in a labyrinth of dialogue built from your open-ended questions and unfinished sentences.

On the plus side, tracking the regression of your verbal exchanges could be a great tool to use when gauging how close your water is to exploding. The more furrowed the brow on the friend you're talking to, the closer you are to popping. It's surprising you aren't getting billed for their wrinkle creams. Speaking of wrinkles, I think we finally solved the agonizing mystery of why so many of us look twenty-five from the eyes down and two-weeks postmortem from the eyes up.

Why You Talk Pretty No Days

It's true—your brain cells really *are* decreasing (#Googlethatshit). So, not only does it feel like you're losing your mind, you literally are and once again you have only the pregnancy hormones to blame. These chemical tricksters ensure that your former self becomes a stranger to your newly parasitized self. And because there will be no shortage of sleepless nights during this time, you will only aggravate this loopiness. We've all described ourselves as "crazy-tired" before, but you're going to mean it this time. Restless nights will occur for a variety of reasons, i.e., being too ~~big~~ blessed to get comfortable or too orally lubricated (it's that excess spit issue again). Being tired helps nobody, and being tired *and* incoherent makes getting through the day extra grueling. We should know. Baby Brain has many of the same symptoms as a hangover, and let us tell you the number of hangovers between us would give even Mel Gibson a run for his money. And just as none of us enjoy the post-drinking haze, we're guessing you aren't head over heels for your sudden aversion to straight-thinking. No one likes to sound as if they belong in a corner and under a dunce cap, but no matter how hard you close your eyes, you cannot close your ears (although you're going to wish you could, especially when junior arrives).

Tips for Keeping It All Together

Try combatting this syndrome as soon as possible, or as soon as you notice everyone around you doubting your intellectual capacities. Onlookers (on*listeners*?) might humor themselves at your expense, but they can also help you stay on top of, well, you. It may be a losing battle, but it's not lost yet, so here are a few tips to kickstart your kickback against yourself:

- *Vitamins for the mind*: omega-3 fatty acids are meant to jog your mental dexterity. But what does that *3* even mean? If it's a measurement of strength, then someone ought to break out the Omega-100s.
- *Writing things down*: here's another chance for you to hone your list-making skills. If you're not a fan of longhand, or if your excess finger weight is making it hard for you to wrangle a pen, you

can always record the important things on your mobile device. A pregnant woman's smartphone should be 90 percent voice memos and 10 percent low battery. Let's face it, none of us know how to keep a phone charged.

- Hypnotism: It's been reported that Jimmy Kimmel's best friend, Matt Damon, quit smoking through sessions of hypnotism. First of all, *as if*, and second of all, if this really works and you *can* have your control panel reconfigured to weaken the baby brain woes, wouldn't that be great? Your friends can get in on the action too and have their hypnotist get to the bottom of why they care so much about your pregnancy in the first place. How do you like them apples?

Everyone Laughs ~~at~~ With the Pregnant Lady

Someone pointed out that along with trying to see the bright side of Momnesia, an expectant woman should take pleasure in her "small triumphs." After reading up on that a bit further, we quickly realized that the "triumphs" in question were *so* minor they would barely pass as accomplishments—things like "remembering to move a load of laundry from the washer to the dryer" or "understanding how to use your breast pump without its instructions." This, readers, is what you call "reaching."

By all means applaud yourself but, for god's sake, dare to aspire for more. You shouldn't have to hear multiple "congratulations" for the completion of menial tasks. It's patronizing, in the same way that it's patronizing whenever one is handed a medal for participation. So, if any of your friends try to tell you (best intentions or not) that knowing how to operate your breast pump makes up for forgetting how to pronounce your last name, shoot daggers. Nobody should be undermining your intelligence, even when your intelligence is undermining itself.

Having a baby on the way can be befuddling, no ifs, ands, or buts about it, and one of your main objectives should be to put whatever is left of your mind at ease. As long as you know that you're doing the best you can, you'll be able to keep on trucking. Even when you misplace the keys.

CRAVINGS AND HANGER

You Weren't a Great Cook Then, and You Sure as Hell Don't Know What You're Doing Now

Hanger doesn't discriminate, so why is it only pregnant women who get their cravings indulged by pretty much anyone, at pretty much any time? What about the rest of the women all over the world—the ones who are getting their periods or the ones who are fetus-free for the time being, or the ones on an all-night bender? Don't we all deserve a Big Mac at midnight if the mood should strike? The answer is yes. Yes, *of course* we do.

Cravings come on strong and fast, like desperately horny men at last call and are similarly hard to shake. However, unlike the boys foraging around the club at closing time, hanger pangs cannot be "cockblocked" with a series of slurred insults or a vodka drink to the face. They are impossibly persistent, and they won't just "move along" or "go home" or "fuck off."

Prepare for your taste buds, as you have always known them, to forsake you. What would normally be a run-of-the-mill pickle craving pre-pregnancy might become garlic dills on a bed of ice cream (Britney Spears fessed up to this one). Maybe you're dying for lasagna . . . on mac'n'cheese or Shepherd's pie) for a light mid-morning nibble, or a simple Turducken for your afternoon commute. Maybe you'll forget what you hate, forget you're a vegetarian (if you are), forget you eat kosher (if you do), or, just like Kourtney Kardashian, forget that relish and mayonnaise should never meet between two slices of bread.

That's what the maternal condition does: it throws you into a culinary Bizarro World where everything is backward and peculiar. These shifts in dietary demands can be one hell of an inconvenience to satisfy, and the burden of your completely counterintuitive menu will land squarely on your partner (or whoever you look to for help in general). There is no beaten path for them to follow, no way for them to stay one step ahead of your requests. If it makes you feel better, express your apologies and gratitude to the friends and loved ones who will accommodate you during this period—feeding pregnant women is a massive pain in the ass.

Food for Fraught

There is an entirely bunk (yet still mega-perpetuated) idea that moms-to-be can eat whatever they want without consequence. Granted, it would be a much-deserved blessing for a gender whose alimental cravings are routinely stifled by the judgments of the patriarchy. Unfortunately, it doesn't work that way. Doctors, being the buzzkills that they are (a flaw we will discuss in a later chapter), will advise you to "eat healthy" and "practice moderation." Some days, you'll listen to them; others, you'll pretend you're starring in your own romantic comedy, elbow-deep into your second gallon of Ben & Jerry's. But no matter how isolating the pregnancy, do not let cabin fever convince you you're Bridget Jones. You are *not*.

The ice-cream frenzy, however, is real. An article from the Journal of the American Dietetic Association found that in the United States, pregnant women are most commonly on the hunt to satisfy a sweet tooth—this means anyone looking to validate their cuddle sessions with frozen dairy now has the professionally backed "go-ahead" they've been waiting for. So, indulge with reckless abandon. Stock the fridge with chocolate chips and Klondike bars. Science says it's cool, and since women are natural people pleasers, we really don't have a choice.

Your newfound confectionary wealth will bring all your friends "to the yard." And while we're on the subject of snacking, is anyone else picking up on these parallels—do the sloppy spoils of the pregnant women more than somewhat resemble those of the woman scorned? This whole chapter basically describes every newly single woman's nutritional needs. Except the maternal diet isn't one driven by self-pity and powerless rage. It's driven by friends and family. To the store. To grab whatever the hell you want, as long as it's not alcohol.

When "Eat Dirt!" Becomes ". . . *Eat Dirt?*"

Researchers posit that this behavior may be the body's complicated way of telling you you're low on something it needs, though it's not usually clear what it is. Hmmm, ambiguous signals in the search for resolve . . . that sounds about right. Your body *is* a woman after all (and so are ours, so we can make jokes like that). If this is the case, scientists should drop whatever it is they're doing and establish a conversion chart. Women don't want to know *why* they're indulging; they want to know *what* to do about it. For instance, say you're peckish for a stick of pepperoni wrapped in cheese slices dipped in jam—a quick glance at the chart might instead steer you toward two bananas, saving you from forever ruining cylindrical meats—best of all shaped meats.

Such a chart would come in handy, and not just for those who are expecting. Fact: you don't have to be in the family way to find yourself in the middle of a shockingly repulsive meal. Jillian has, twice, been caught eating from her sister's compost, and she swears to god that both of those times she thought it was a salad. With a conversion system in place, Jillian could finally work through her mysterious inclination for decaying organic material (an issue the chart would likely equate to a psychiatric appointment), and moms and non-moms alike could explore their cravings openly, including the reportedly common urge to bury spades of soil or dirt down their gullets (soil cravings are a thing; there is even a word for it: *geophagy*).

Let You Eat Cake

The truth is nobody finds your weird appetite repugnant. It's the palpable envy that's making everyone sick. Who wouldn't want to eat whatever, whenever, and be able to hide all the evidence behind a growing baby? They say the grass is always greener on the other side, and in this case, this grass is edible and pregnant women are mowing down as if they were Christian Slater hoovering caviar at Ted Danson's house (*Curb Your Enthusiasm*, "Hot Towel").

Chow down on whatever is in front of you. With a shit storm on the horizon, you deserve for everyone to keep their mouths shut so you can carry on with your feast. Crumble those Doritos into your ravioli! Spoil yourself with whatever stomach-churning creations you have jammed up your tightening sleeves. They're likely made of some sort of elastic material and can spare the room.

MATERNITY WEAR

Maternity Pants Are Hilarious,
and Everyone Wants Five Pairs

There's no way getting around this one. Biggie sizing your fries is a real temptation, but when it comes to upsizing our wardrobes, we get upset. As much as you'll want to fight against your expansion, your little juggernaut's determination to grow will fight back even harder —and it will win. He or she now calls the shots, flexing a propensity for selfishness like a seasoned pro (a quality that only strengthens with age, as adulthood will testify). Resistance, as they say, is futile.

Babies won't wait for you to prepare yourself for that moment when you can no longer see your feet or feel contrition when you are forced to abandon your pelvic landscaping routine (see chapter 3). They don't give a shit about your old jeans and how they made your ass look before you graduated to new pairs; those jeans won't be making it back into the regular rotation for a long while anyhow. In fact, none of your go-to pieces will. Replacing your old clothes with current maternity options (in an economically friendly way) is about as easy as trying to find a Donna Karan Needle Punch in a haystack of adult-sized Cabbage Patch Kids clothing.

Trying on clothes is always a touchy subject, regardless of one's uterine disposition. Big, small, slight, round; we've all stood horrified in front of our mirrors, clinging to the belt-loops that have been stretched to the point of near severance after one-too-many failed attempts at pulling our pants up and over our thighs. But these knee-jerk bad feelings brought upon by wardrobe malfunctions can be mitigated with humor. When *you* can laugh at yourself, it means *friends* can laugh at you, too, and laughing *with* someone is much more acceptable than laughing *at* someone—or so we have all been told.

It's nothing personal. Seeing a woman struggle with zippers while trying to keep one's boobs in check is enough to set anybody off. Not because people are insensitive to your emotional well-being, but because bodies are funny! Consider what your pals' empathy is up against: elastic waistbands, piles of empire-waisted tops, hand-me-down overalls, and maternity fashion that resembles adult lines of Osh Kosh B'Gosh.

We promise that your self-esteem will overcome this beating. But it won't be easy. At least these next few paragraphs will help you clothe your baby belly and save you from the self-enforced reclusion we know you've been considering.

Dressing Up . . . in Style?

Whenever we are feeling especially bloated, we always look for the tarp-iest tops and bottoms to accommodate our ballooning. In a perfect world, we imagine ourselves styling our duvet as a cocoon and climbing inside for the duration of the metamorphosis—whether it be menses or pregnancy—sans social condemnation, sans the constrictions of non-stretch fabrics. When going out to restaurants, enjoying family get-togethers, or sipping coffee in hipster-pretentious cafes, decked in roomy modesty cloaks, free to be their authentic, incubatory selves. If you're having trouble building a visual reference, a similar look was featured in Disney's *The Little Mermaid*. Not the pink dress she wore to dinner but the horror she wore when she got first transformed. All bound by rope, she sashayed around Prince Eric's backyard—we mean, beach—acting like God's gift. That's the look. Even though Ariel decided to ensconce herself in canvas as opposed to cotton, it was obvious by her styling choices that she was pregnant or perhaps riding the crimson wave—and what better way to do so than by donning a sail.

It's okay to secretly wish for a similar Disney-inspired pregnancy body bag, but we cannot help wonder why women fantasize about hiding underneath unspeakable garments whenever we slip outside our BMI comfort zone? When did we decide that looking as if we've completely given up on ourselves was a more desirable option than showcasing a little paunch every now and then? It seems we've been conditioned to see gaining weight (whether water- or baby-based) a fate much worse than looking stupid.

It doesn't help that maternity-wear designers seem to base every outfit on the theory that as the client expands, so should the silhouette. By that logic, any woman who has reached her point of popping will be dressed in a glorified eight-man tent, creating the risk of hospital waiting areas being confused for overbooked state parks. And that's not good for anybody.

In the Words of De La Soul: It *Ain't* All Good

We have seen some marketing slogans trying to convince pregnant women that modern maternity attire is no longer the hideous parasitic twins of your regular wardrobe. This begs two questions: "Who are they kidding?" and "Says who?" The areas of the body most impacted by a successfully fertilized egg are generally below the eyes, and not the eyes themselves. Why do these companies continue to crank out collections that rely on the hope that knocked-up women will generally have bad taste in clothes? Sure, there have been improvements, but maternity wear has a well-documented history of being categorically unflattering, and any claims that the missteps are behind us are at the very least a stretch and at the very most an all-out lie.

Maternity Puns Are Not Okay

During your pregnancy, T-shirts are something you can, and should, wear the bejesus out of. These anchor pieces go with absolutely anything and look super cute pulled over a baby belly. V-neck, boatneck, scoop neck; red, navy, stripes, florals, polka-dots. Work each and every one you own. You don't have to overthink anything when you wear a T-shirt, except for this—no words allowed, specifically, no maternity puns.

For the first few months, pregnant women live with the constant fear of judgment—fear that their community suspects they are putting on pounds for reasons other than getting knocked up. Every socially adept person understands that it's totally unacceptable to ask a woman if she is carrying a baby, so those not in the know are often left piecing together the clues on their own. This can be a recipe for the worst kind of disaster when people, well intentioned or not, jump to the wrong conclusions and put their feet so far down their throats they are able to kick their own ass. To skirt the uncertainty, someone decided that qualification via comedy, i.e., printing pregnancy puns on T-shirts, was the only solution—and none of us are laughing.

Think "Pregasaurus Rex" or "I'm making a human, what have you have done today?" A picture of an un-zipped zipper revealing a cartoon infant peeking from within, with a speech bubble floating out from its mouth: "Hiding until due date"; "Peek-a-boo!"; or "Let me out!" These are just a few of the garish designs that have been spotted on individuals under the influence of pregnancy. These are bad. Really, really bad, and, in our view, they demonstrate two things: 1. We don't find the same things funny. 2. People are *desperate* for the public acknowledgment of their unborn child.

After reading a shirt's message, friends, family, and strangers are suddenly thrown into a conversation to which they might not have consented. Now they are expected to ask probing questions like "How far along are you?" or else *they're* the asshole. It's a stunning example of passive-obnoxious behavior on the mom-to-be's part, and unluckily for everyone, there is an endless supply of these "punny" articles of clothing. But if you like kitsch and you're still on the fence as to who is right and who is wrong in this debate ("Pregasaurus

Rex" alone should have put the argument to bed), consult the wit below and don't be shocked when you find yourself wondering if some women aren't getting pregnant for the exact same reason *Seinfeld*'s Tim Whatley converted to Judaism: the jokes.

- "Miracle in Progress" (A cue to vomit?)
- "It's His Fault ➔" (We get it. That's your partner. Relax.)
- "If I'm related to these people, I'm not coming out . . ." (Already the mom is speaking for her child.)
- "Baby Loading . . . Please Wait" (Computers are so funny.)
- "Birth Control is for Sissies" (This wasn't a gift from her parents.)
- "We're hoping it's a Dinosaur" (What does that even mean?)
- "The baby made me eat it" (Did the baby make you eat the whole box?)
- "Pregnant is the new skinny" (It's really not.)
- "I humped, now I'm bumped" (The word *humping* is cancelled.)
- "Don't eat Watermelon Seeds" (Is there any space left on the sign-up sheet for that mission to Mars?)

Seth Cohen was right—"big funny" is the pits. Shirts that announce the sex. Shirts that announce the due date. Friends shouldn't let friends wear . . . whatever *this* is, so if you're heading toward this kind of maternity styling, be ready for your BFFs to come at you with some tough love. Your clothes aren't meant to be your voice; that's what your voice is for. We don't care if it's "Calvin Klein" or "I ♥ My Bump"; the risk is too great during this critical fashion period. Avoid them like the Whos avoid the Grinch with that infamous "thirty-nine-and-a-half-foot pole" we hear so much about every Christmas. Sounds like a pretty safe distance to us.

Expandable Wear

Some designers may have left their thinking caps on a little too long. In valiant attempts to accommodate evolving pregnancy bodies, while still being low-maintenance, pieces have begun to emerge that can move through trimesters *without* you needing to upsize. Imagine a dress with fabric packed and folded into the mid-section with origami-like precision that, like an accordion, expands and contracts as you do. A practical answer to impractical size issues. Regrettably, the aesthetics don't favor real-life settings (AKA, society) and it would take a very particular type of women to throw something so "avant garde" into her shopping cart. You know the ones—they're the vegans with finicky glasses; they're reading books on attachment parenting; they have the kinds of bicycles with billy-goat horned handles, and they wear boxy linen vests with one big wooden button in the middle. Have we made enough generalizations yet?

Maybe you disagree that convertible clothing has a certain type of woman, but can we at least agree it has a certain type of environment? Take the set of the TV show *The 100*, for instance, where a group of post-apocalyptic survivors wear clothes in various states of disrepair (even when their hair is perfectly blown out and their makeup professionally touched up). Each character in the series is damned to don the same get-up every day because that's what happens when you're trapped on Earth in the wake of nuclear devastation—nobody is carrying around a change of clothes. This is the perfect scenario for a maternity dress that accommodates your bump in real-time. However, since most of us have the privilege of taking our clothes off at the end of the day, we don't really need this (unless we're lazy or plan to invest in as few pieces of maternity wear as possible).

Still, trying to make things easier for the pregnant lady is a lovely gesture. There are worse crimes than looking like you plan on being stranded at an airport for the next nine months, luggage lost, wearing the only garment that will fit you for the next forty weeks as a preventive measure. And whether you're itching to try items from the expandable line or you're not, remember that we're still living pre-apocalypse.

Misguided Designs

When one thinks of bad maternity wear, it's never without flashes of the teachers who came in and out of our lives during elementary school wearing clown-sized dungarees, bibbed dresses, sailor-themed jumpsuits, and cap sleeves upon cap sleeves upon cap sleeves. Before the turn of the millennium, many women were encouraged to downplay their baby bumps and cover up—at least that's what their clothing suggested. When comparing these dated looks to today's "contemporary" selections, not much has changed. Oversized bows paired with sashes or any other type of material that can be tied are trends that are still going strong. In fact, there seems to be a reoccurring theme among designers to bind up pregnant women like they were securing a mattress to a car's roof rack to ensure safe passage. By this stage, most of you already feel like a minivan anyway, so it was only a matter of time before somebody took it upon themselves to dress you as such.

Then there's the empire waist/short-sleeve duo. This remains a heavy hitter in the mommy-to-be world, and it leaves us wondering *why*. Maybe it has to do with the belief that the appearance of the arms does not vary *too* noticeably across a pregnancy, and so they end up being exhaustedly highlighted. Whatever the reason, the result is oddly juvenile and only suitable for women ready to go up against your 1990s Polly Pocket in a "Who Wore It Best?" contest—and lose. All these cutesy bits might work on a Teacup Yorkie, but not on any of the pregnant women we know. They are far less innocent and much more mature than a cap sleeve implies; they're pregnant, for Christ's sake! They get busy, and they aren't afraid to show it! So, let's see some cleave! But, first, let's talk about pants.

Maternity Pants Are Everyone's Spirit Animal

They are bewitching. You won't believe how freeing the concept is—the look of jeans with the forgiveness of elastic, and *not* one of the scrunchy, conspicuous waistbands we all know and hate—unless you're a hipster, in which case you consider the bulky, baggy, elastic waistline very *en vogue*. In fact, you might as well skip this whole chapter as we assume you've already been shopping in the maternity section for some time now.

These pants seduce you through their sheer unseductiveness. These roomy babies enrapture, and their allure goes far beyond the maternal clientele. They speak the language of every woman—the one who frequents the all-you-can-eat Chinese buffet, the one who never refuses seconds or thirds at a turkey dinner, or the one who dabbles in substantial amounts of weekday or weekend beer drinking. Forget loosening belt buckles or releasing buttons—maternity pants provide one uber-wide forgivable band that can comfortably bend to the will of any spare tire. It's the dreamboat your waist down has been waiting to travel in, so don't be surprised if friends ask to try yours on, whether it be for shits and giggles or driven by genuine intrigue. It proves there are still those who want to "get into your pants," even if it is just a couple of women you've known forever.

Clothes Are Just That—Clothes

Not being able to wear what you want or look the way you're accustomed to looking requires a deep adjustment and can cause you to become discouraged. But here's why you shouldn't listen to your unforgiving self-perception: This clothes issue is a small thing that just happens to come in a large size. It will get easier, and it *will* get funnier even if you can't see the humor in it now (you will once it's all over). Every terrible, awful, no-good experience will become an anecdote kept in your back pocket for whenever you need to slay a room. That's pretty powerful stuff, like ring-of-Mordor power-ful—one elastic waistband to rule them all, one elastic waistband to bind them.

HOME & NATURAL VS. HOSPITALS & THE GOOD DRUGS

In the Words of Charlotte York:
"I Choose My Choice"

Before a woman becomes pregnant, it's likely she has already envisioned where she will be having her baby. Allison gave birth at the infirmary, surrounded by chaos and a series of "WTF" moments. When Jillian pictures herself giving birth, she sees panic, tears, blood, guts, epidural needles, and speaking in tongues. She imagines the sterile walls of a hospital room, and men and women in scrubs who went above and beyond protocol by spending the last two days washing their hands. This means, should her water ever break, it's off to the maternity ward like Allison had done so before her, as opposed to, say, her living room, to slip into the birthing pool she will never buy.

But hey, that's only one way of doing it. The other method is the more "organic" route, away from the interventions of modern medicine. The question is how do you know which is for you? Debates between home versus hospital and natural versus loopy (?) deliveries have gained serious traction over the last few decades. And things have gotten *pretty* hostile. Women, especially those who have lived the experience, draw hard lines and hurl accusations against one another, ignoring the obvious fact that everyone is different and that, therefore, every woman's birthing needs will be met through different methods.

Could this be another example of Mom Brain rearing its ugly head? There's no way to be sure, just like, there's no objective winner in these battles. Each has its own success stories (i.e., the stuff you *don't* hear about) and, more notably, its own sensationalized stories (i.e., the stuff you *do* hear about). Think of it this way: no one ever writes a 1,200-word review when they enjoy themselves at a restaurant. But a waiter gives Jillian a "look" when she orders gravy? Says they only have something called an "au jus," and when she says, "Sure, fine, whatever," they return to inform her they really only serve "demi-jus"? Well, one thing is for sure: she is opening her laptop as soon as she gets home to let the world know that said establishment must be trolled and destroyed. And that's like what happens here. Sort of . . .

Women love to "warn." They are "warners," and these warnings come in many forms and from many more directions. Even with all the do's and dont's stuffing up the atmosphere, it's hard to say definitively which birthing method will be the better, more responsible choice for you. And that's what reconnaissance is for. Make sure that a) you know all the options available to you, and b) your family and friends are actually informed before you listen to anything they say. There's a big difference between those who know what they're talking about and those who *think* they know what their talking about, and if you plan to accept outsiders into your deliberation process, you need to be able to spot the difference. With that said, this chapter shouldn't be anyone's bible, but it can be their starting point.

Home Births

It wasn't too long ago when those going against the grain were getting all the side-eye. Most of the parenting world used to be quite comfortable maligning the home birthing method to the hippies and love-zombies of our society. Here's a head's up—the times? They are *still* a changing. There has been a shift in social norms. Again. Would you believe that more and more "regular" people are choosing home-birthing over hospital stays? Plebes like us, and maybe even you?

It's true! Even celebrities (that's right, *celebrities*) are climbing on board. And if planned effectively, these births are safer than ever. If you consider yourself a woman who likes to appear ahead of her time, or if you're looking to "keep up with the Joneses," you should know that the Joneses are probably having their babies at home now. If you want in on the in-crowd, or are simply too lazy to get your ass to the local infirmary, this is a good, doable choice. Just don't get crazy and try to go at it alone; it's not intended to be a solo event. It doesn't matter who you are, or how much you think you know—this procedure requires *a lot* of guidance. Now, let's see who you will be teaming up with.

The Doula: The Emotional Acolyte

Not to be confused with the midwife, the doula is sort of like the "one to watch" in terms of home births. Sure, they've been on the scene forever, but they have only recently been getting the attention they deserve. Unfortunately, there are still those who associate the d-word with some unfavorable stereotypes.

For starters, let's look at the word itself: *doula*. It feels a little like crunchy granola in the mouth, and when it to comes to something as physically traumatic as childbirth, most people choose to rely on individuals whose job titles end in "-ologist" or "-trician" (as opposed to the sound we imagine escapes the lips of a French man post-orgasm). Also, not to add fuel to the fire, Jillian's sister asserts that some doulas don't have any children of their own (phonies!). Then again, in almost the same accusatory breath, she revealed the other side of that coin, which is that many of them in fact *do*. So, although we gained nothing from that particular conversation, and you gained nothing from our mentioning of it, it's a perfect segue to our unreasonably negative list of the preconceived notions surrounding these birthing assistants:

- Doulas are vegans carrying plant-based propaganda in ugly purses.
- Doulas sing "Happy Birthday" in their best voice.
- Doulas are the ones who hug the person holding a "Free Hugs" sign.
- Doulas are always rolling their eyes at men.
- Doulas don't buy or wear pants that are long enough in the inseam.
- Doulas will ask someone in passing how they're doing and *mean* it.
- During delivery, doulas want midwives to shut up, and vice versa.

We're going to stick by the vegan one (just because we like to get under people's skin), but the rest of these observations are totally without cause. The true role of a doula is to emotionally guide a woman through her pre- and post-natal periods and to serve as her advocate. Sure, they have about as much medical training as any- one who *doesn't* have medical training, but clinical work is not their intention. If you have questions, they have the answers. And if they don't, they find the answers so you don't have to. Doulas will give the evil eye to your partner when you cannot muster the energy and will verbally bitch slap a medical profesh should they stray away from your finely tuned birth plan.

In a super touchy-feely nutshell, doulas are there to add to your army—an unconditional back-haver. If you're nervous, experiencing wavering confidence, or feeling incapable, you may want to consider seeking out one of these badass bitches. There's nothing wrong with adding one more to your corner, and the doula just may be the cheerleader you have been missing.

Midwife: The Rebel

In America and Canada, under the North American Registry of Midwives, you can enter a three-year pro- gram to become a certified professional midwife (CPM). They are educated and have framed pieces of paper to prove it. But still, despite their legitimate training, they continue to be hounded by their own unfair, though somewhat comical, stigmas.

If you haven't already seen the entirety of *The Mindy Project*, we'll assume you do what most of us do when we're behind (or uninterested) in the show everyone's talking about and pretend that you've seen it. Either way, you're likely aware of the sitcom's midwife representatives, Brendan and Duncan Deslaurier, who enter the series accused of stealing patients from Mindy and her colleagues. The show's writers hit all the damaging labels that commonly surround midwifery (pronounced *mid-whiff-fer-ree*, making it our new favorite word), and the holistic duo unleash their counterattacks. The resulting episodes are the perfect blend of rib-tickling rhetoric and shallow bickering, the kind you would expect from these two disciplines meeting in the exaggerated version of "real life" that is television. Truthfully, the brothers might be the best part of the whole series, which is great because it puts mid-whiff-fer-fee squarely in the middle of popular culture. And not a moment too soon, because by the time you get through this rap sheet of (fictitious) transgressions, you'll agree they could use a win:

- Midwives are usually too tall and look like they would be good at volleyball.

- Midwives wear power suits made with scrub materials and corrective footwear.
- Midwives are vegetarians.
- Midwives have feminist ulterior motives.
- Midwives wear French braids.
- Midwives hope you will make the right choice and home-school.
- Midwives are women (God, no!).

And those are just off the top of our heads. Again, this list may loosely describe *one* midwife we know, but it in no way reflects on the profession as a whole. Our bullet points are 100 percent bogus, *especially* that last one, because in 2013, Otis Kryzanauskas was acknowledged as one out of the more-than-thousand registered midwives in the Canadian Association of Midwives. Or should we say midhusband? Either way, what a privilege for us women to see a man break through that one remaining barrier, and being Canucks ourselves, we applaud Otis for making the CAM gender-diverse and whatever the opposite of a "sausage party" is . . .

Midwives are more than equipped to deal with regular birth circumstances outside of a medical facility (though they can make an appearance inside one, as well). If you plan on staying home for the whole shebang, for god's sake make sure you have one of these broads (or bros) on hand. It takes guts (sometimes literally) to try for the unaided home birth, and getting through it on your own or with your plus-one doula is rarely going to cut it. It sometimes takes a little bit more than a series of "way to go's," breathing exercises, and advantageous birthing positions to deliver a baby. Empowering words cannot monitor a baby's heart rate or cut an umbilical cord. A midwife can do both things and more. She or he can take you from mother-to-be to mother-that-be status, and if things do go haywire (god forbid), you can rely on a midwife to make the tough calls ... to the ambulance.

To summarize, the doula is there for comfort and peace of mind, to inspire you to push out that baby and not give up. A midwife is there to make sure that both mother and baby pull through in a safe and stable condition. When these two operate in tandem, they make one hell of a team.

Doctors: the New Underdog?

Some say that women have the least control over their delivery if they decide to check into the hospital. Medical professionals have tried and tested methods they feel benefit the majority. They may be able to deviate from these methods on a case-by-case basis, but when you're in that delivery room, the doctor knows best, not you.

This doesn't leave much room for a personalized experience you would have in a planned home birth, where time and attention are laid on thick and heavy. Hospitals, like restaurants, are all about success and turnover, so chances are once you settle in and have your cut-and-dry birth, they'll be prepping you to settle out.

However brief and distancing, these practices used to be taken as gospel and were rarely questioned; but that was then, and this is now. Today, women are taking back the delivery room, and doctors are starting to feel the sting, their more unassuming colleagues have been dealing with for years. But how could anyone fault the selfless altruism of the med-school grad, you ask? Here are a few things that come to mind when the evil OB-GYN is on the brain:

- Doctors eat meat for sadistic pleasure.
- Doctors think they're better than doulas and midwives.
- Doctors always let their latex gloves snap dramatically to demonstrate power.
- Doctors wish they had Google Glass, if they don't already, and they own many unnecessarily flashy gadgets.
- Doctors get their shoes shined in airports like assholes.

- Doctors get into obstetrics for the fanfare and to satiate their god complex.
- Women and men everywhere want to date doctors.

Google Glass? It's just so showy. Whatever happened to behaving like a humble human being and getting your glasses from the Dollar Store like the rest of us posers (Jillian has three pairs, one for each of her zero prescriptions)? These exaggerations are not indicative of incompetence, but mainly of someone who is drowning in arrogance. In this context, though, arrogance may be exactly what someone rattled by the idea of childbirth needs. Staying home isn't for softies, and giving birth to a child one way or the other won't earn you any medals, though you might have thought otherwise the way some women talk about skipping their epidurals. You know what? Stop telling people for years to come that you didn't have one. Coming from our most inoffensive of places, no one cares.

Zapping the pain with the prick of a needle does not make you any less mighty of a child-bearer. Those who commit themselves months before to forgoing the procedure have been known to renege. Even if you have a doula or midwife with you in hospital, an epidural administered by an anesthesiologist is on the table. And if people rag on you for going with traditional western medicine, then allow us to share one of our favorite go-to mantras: *Fuck 'em.* This is not one of those situations where you should bend to peer pressure or where the opinions of others matter. You should be consulting facts, books, and peer-reviewed journals, not biased judgments or malarkey attached to bullet points. Do not confuse show-offs for savants or satire for truth. Not only is laughter *not* "the best medicine," it's also not the best source, either.

So ... Then What?

In the end, it's up to parents to decide which way they will go. But honestly, it's also up to the ultrasound. The baby's progression and health are considerations that are much more valid in this decision than anyone's principles. And isn't the former what's most important when six to ten pounds of your temporary insides are being "ectomy-ed"? Following one's moral compass sounds ideal, but minimizing risk should always come before your preferred choice of delivery. No matter where you end up, whether it be on all fours in your bed or spread-eagle on a gurney, there will always be enough judgment to go around, so there's no point in sweating it. Not only should you not try to please everyone, you very literally can't and won't.

SECTION 3
THE THIRD TRIMESTER

THE BABY SHOWER

Everyone Hates a Baby Shower

You have hit the third trimester. Everything is about to be pushed into overdrive, starting with the dreaded baby shower. Baby showers are a rite of passage for pregnant women across the globe. They are the "party" method of reminding friends who is (and who *isn't*) about to have a baby (in case anyone managed to forget). Baby showers usually involve a sensory onslaught of streamers, buntings, balloons, and towers of gift bags choking on blue or pink tissue paper. Basically, picture what a six-year-old's birthday might look like if he or she were to have their own Platinum Visa, or the scene that might unfold if the Dollar General were to blow up and you catered the wreckage with finger foods and mimosas.

These days, the celebrations are on a downswing, suffering from a bit of a bad rap due to their frivolous nature. Everyone seems to have lost their sense of humor when it comes to eating melted chocolate out of diapers or playing "guess the baby food" (chicken and gravy, anyone?). It's a shame, really, because there *is* good stuff at the core of your pregnancy; you just need the right friend to flaunt it for you. Someone who is ready and able to take on the task, someone to help baby showers find their "it" factor again, and someone who is willing to shove their face into a pair of diapers in the quest to discover if it's a melted Hershey bar they're tasting or if they got the one filled with actual shit (that's how the game works, right?).

The Guest of Honor

Because baby showers aren't making moms-to-be weak in the cankles the way they used to, it's become completely acceptable for some women to refuse them altogether. But don't assume you're off the hook. You may recoil at the thought of being the focal point of a large group, especially when you're feeling like a grounded blimp, but if you skip out on this revelry, you may regret it. The truth is, the sooner you realize that passing on something just because it *might* be terrible could mean passing on an opportunity to add something new to your list of things to complain about—like prenatal yoga or taking the stairs—the sooner the FOMO can take hold. Nothing makes a woman buckle and cave like a healthy dose of FOMO. We're still saying *FOMO*, right?

Let gal pals know exactly what parts of the event you find particularly vapid, and why. There's nothing wrong with butchering tradition if it means getting you into the spirit. Do the games make you squeamish? Then kibosh the games. If it's a forced belly casting session you dread, give friends permission to hurt anyone trying to sneak a plaster kit onto the premises. Drop every "iffy" activity like Ken dropped Barbie once that saucy Midge came strolling down Barbie Lane (nineties kids know who we're talking about), and threaten any guest bold enough to suggest that things proceed otherwise. Good friends are never afraid to take a bitch or two out. What the guest of honor wants, the guest of honor gets.

Hosting Duties

Regardless of who stakes their claim in the planning and organizing, you'll want to maintain some, but not too much, involvement. Baby showers are someone else's problem, not yours, which is perhaps their only redeeming quality. If your mom or sister(s) want the reins, let friends know so they can hand them over and never look back. Though it's true many of us love to steer these sorts of ships, there are also those who appreciate being looked over. It's not like anyone is getting cut out completely—there are still seats on the party bus; they just won't be driving (which means they can drink!).

If you're afraid of offending the go-getters and planners of your group by withholding hosting titles, remind them that when they're not hosting, obligations are downgraded extensively. Responsibilities go from picking up champagne, food, and decorations to simply picking up after the guests—or if it's a co-ed party, maybe just "picking up." Regular guests can simply back away from any impending disasters (i.e., not enough variation in chip flavor or too few balloons) and join in the verbal tirade when you inevitably begin to criticize.

Hosting *anything* can be hell. You're essentially asking somebody to give their living space a rigorous and socially acceptable clean (which sucks) *and* spend some of their pretty pennies (side note: adults do not require gift bags). Hellish or not, these downsides will forever be rolled with because most good friends are, first and foremost, good people who should probably get up off their asses and clean their homes anyway, however begrudgingly.

The Location

Wherever your host calls home is usually the easiest place in which to lay your scene. It's not necessarily the best place but certainly the most popular and one that requires the least amount of organization. Those extending their search outside their personal territories should start by exploring the spatial limits of their community—think restaurants, community halls, churches, hotel suites, and clubhouses.

Let's take another look at that last option, because it's a little confusing. For many folks, when you take the word "clubhouse" out of the sandwich section of a menu, you also take it out of its best-known context. Where we come from, when not talking comfort food, clubhouses were places where the family you babysat for drank way too much after golfing eighteen holes or where middle school riffraff would meet to look at stolen *Playboy* magazines and plot hairbrained schemes against their teachers. We're guessing the women reading this aren't running in the same circles as pre-pubescent perverts, so if your ideal baby shower setting is a clubhouse, it's probably the kind that comes with a membership fee, and you should forward any further inquiries over to the token rich girl we all keep on reserve.

Wherever you end up, you better hope it's convenient for you and your invites. Seriously, if a long drive is required, or more than one flight of stairs, go back to the drawing board. While you're at it, ensure that the venue size is proportional to the guest list. It's not a funeral (unless you consider your laying to rest next year's social life), and people shouldn't be expected to stand outside during the "ceremony" because someone doesn't understand the meaning of "maximum capacity." Packed spaces aggravate crowds and can trigger mass "attitude attacks," leading to a *very* bitchy mutiny. Then again, a more realistic possibility is none of this happening at all, though it's still a good practice not to fill the house.

Eeny-Meeny-Miny-Moe

Creating a guest list that neither insults nor excludes is like trying to navigate a minefield—if the mines were a bunch of petulant friends hypersensitive to any sort of ill-perceived personal slight. Think of all the pockets of social circles you have to comb through: the inner circle, outer circle, work circle, family circle, etc. That's a lot of people's days to make, and a lot of hearts to break. Friends who are co-managing the invite list will get an insight to the background operations—seeing who *doesn't* make the final cut is always much juicer than seeing who does. It's quite literally the on-paper division between those with whom you honestly enjoy spending time with and those for whom you may have just been faking it.

Trying to make everyone happy is fatiguing, so if you find yourself wrapped up in finalizations or if you become too concerned about the feelings of others, get someone else to finish your dirty work. Nobody has to notify the non-invited, but slighted individuals will be on the lookout for someone to point the finger at, and this time around it won't be you. You're not in charge (technically), so you can claim complete ignorance and duck all the consequent chin-wag. It's also one of those rare situations where throwing a friend under the bus is a mutual decision. Everyone knows *playing* the asshole is a whole lot easier than *being* the asshole, so don't worry for one second that your appointed scapegoat will be bothered by the potential blowback. Antagonizing disingenuous women, frenemies or not, is oddly delicious.

There is a chance that downsizing your baby shower party will work itself out naturally. If co-workers offer up a separate work shindig, you can reduce the guest list by shaving away the professional fat. Another way to shrink numbers is by throwing a smaller gathering just for family friends (which, we all know, is a more inclusive way of saying your mom's friends). This is often organized by a parent and held at their home. The crowd will be older and the topics of conversation will be sleep-inducing, but it gets those obligatory moments with grandmothers, aunts, and other future members of the Red Hat Society out of the way.

Men and Kids

Martha Stewart says the presence of men or kids at a baby shower is dependent on if you're a modernist (in which case, everyone is welcome) or a traditionalist (in which case, you'd rather die). I think old M. Diddy might be overcomplicating things, because, again, what it really boils down to is not whether you're old- or new-school but rather how much food you are willing to further ration away . Typically, when women realize that opening up a guest list means less nibbles to go around, they vote against it. Don't flirt with hanger. Best to keep the greedy paws of men and children at home.

Invitations

As far as actual invitations are concerned, anything goes. A Facebook group is easy and efficient. E-vites are quick and offer immediate delivery. Old-fashioned snail mail is the bees' knees for invitees to open. They all get the job done, but if we had to break them down into certain terms, there's only one place to start and end: cost. We have free, free, and not free—one of those things is more expensive than the others. But let us give each option its chance to shine, and you and your friends can decide the winner.

Facebook

This is how you keep a dialogue open with relatively no effort. Facebook leaves paper trails, which means you and your friends can check in on all the RSVPs you're forgetting to track due to your rising disinterest in the whole thing. With a Facebook group, planners can get feedback from guests on the itinerary, as well as suggestions on what should be served, what should be brought, who should be talked about, etc.—all without ever having to physically or verbally reach out to anyone (bonus). This is also a great place for friends to share who is buying what that way, everyone can avoid the uber-embarrassing "Who Gave It Best" moments where you receive two identical breast pumps (one for each boob?).

E-vites vs. Snail Mail

Written invitations sent by post are treasures, but the novelty of the gesture has the lifespan of a fruit fly (side note: fruit flies have very short lifespans). Think of the postage cost and all the addresses someone is going to have to collect (don't panic, it won't be you). And does anyone even remember what a stamp tastes like? Do they even make lickable stamps anymore? As soon as the day comes and goes, those invitations end up in the same place as every other card before it: the trash, right next to the Chinese take-out containers and a variety of empties (some of us are too hungover to recycle *all* the time—okay?)

E-vites are child's play. So easy, in fact, that you and your friends may forget to review before sending, which can lead to some pretty messy consequences. This is a lesson in the importance of proofreading. If someone is accidentally omitted or added, there are going to be problems. Remember, we're dealing with women here—in group form. An oversight like this will either never be forgiven or will be brought up passive-aggressively for the remainder of [insert whoever is responsible]'s life. It's better to practice preventive methods in this situation as opposed to relying on one's ability to do damage control. Whoever is in charge should employ a St. Nicholas–style of due-diligence by checking this list twice.

Decorations

Friends do the decorating. They usually have an idea of what they need but a loose understanding of exactly what to do. Many websites claim that one can never go wrong with keeping it classy, but this advice is boring, and the reasoning behind it may not have anything to do with aesthetics or exercising restraint. We have read that the veto on embellished decorating assumes that it "distracts guests' attention away from the mother." Look it up. This conspiracy theory is very much alive. Now, unless we are decorating someone's home exclusively with tinsel and inviting only cats, this will not be a legitimate concern. Then again, now that we've put it out there, every time you hear anyone pushing party planners to dial it down, you'll always suspect it's simply their way of disguising their selfishness as taste.

Also, be careful: friends aren't mind readers and won't always head in the direction you are pointing. Sometimes they'll opt to be that fun friend, the one that goes all out, balls to the wall. Streamers, balloons, baby straws, baby napkins, and maybe an ice sculpture of the female anatomy. You may be initially horrified, but do not underestimate the great humor in gaudiness. Typically, baby shower color palettes are muted and for the dull and the weak, so appreciate the squad member who's willing to break down the dusty rose and powder blue barriers for something more jolting. For instance, black can really stifle the energy if you're interested in making people uncomfortable. That is obviously an asshole suggestion, but we dare you.

Register for Gifts or No?

This depends on your intentions: do you plan to birth the baby or marry it? A gift is a gift. It's free, it's thoughtful, and whatever it is, it is *not* your decision. Think about your childless friends who don't really spend much time thinking about, let alone shopping for, people who aren't themselves, much less someone who is under the age of zero (unless they're, like, a really good person). Plus, a registry confiscates guests' freedom to freak out as they sashay down the aisles of Toys "R" Us. It spoils the fun and puts a hard emphasis on the F-U. And don't try to convince us that it's a good idea because you'll get some sort of discount on baby items later on in the future. Nice try, lady.

Then again, this isn't about your guests, is it? This is about you, so of *course* it makes sense to make a damn registry (though we're sticking by the sentiments we expressed earlier). There's shit you *actually* need and, as we have suggested, some people won't have the faintest idea what those things are. A registry could have saved Jillian from buying her sister a Christian children's book that went into detail about Jesus and what appeared to be a poor man's version of the Titanic, except with animals. Her family, incidentally, do not identify as "god fearing," but that's what can happen when a clueless person equipped with an inattention for detail shops for a baby—they'll end up with something, but only as long as nobody needs it. So make a registry, or don't make a registry. Ultimately, it's a shower. Some gifts will be what you want, and some gifts will be what you get.

Receiving the Gift

The only thing better than getting gifts is watching a pregnant friend get gifts, and that is not sarcasm. The over-the-top reactions are so *transparent* and so *amazing*—or at least they better be. You cannot afford to offend any of your future babysitters. For a strong game face, we suggest studying Taylor "Sssss"-wift. If there were a Nobel Prize in Artificial Graciousness, she would win it every year. So, when an item is placed in your lap, you gotta smile like you're a top contender. That's how it works—you're handed something, you grin like you should be institutionalized, and then you put that something off to the side or onto the floor, where friends can rummage through without asking or apologizing.

But what will the vultures find in the remains? The contents of these gifts are *not* the sex-y products that often turn up at bridal showers (what point did they become quasi-fantasia parties, anyway?); they're more the sex-*ed* products—think practicality meets the *Where Did I Come From?* movie. For example:

- Bulb syringes: used to suck the snot out of your baby's nose. Or anyone's nose, really.
- Pee pee teepees: Not yet available for the adult male. You put these atop boys' penises to keep

them from peeing onto walls, into faces, or any-where else.

- Breastfeeding covers: Perfect for the modest woman or magician-in-training.
- Belly bands: Probably the only time anyone gets away with giving a woman something that implies she needs to suck in.

Food

Depending on the kind of family you grew up with, the people you surround yourself with, and how pregnant of a person you are, food will be the most important part of the baby shower. Let's face it, food is the most impor-tant part of any event. Females can *eat*. Even those who don't usually eat much always make an exception when the food is free, the company is female, and the bathroom is familiar. You won't be the only one packing in enough for two, just the only one with an excuse. To paraphrase: there better be enough to go around.

Keep it straightforward. Baby-themed treats can be cute, but there's no need for you or your planner to fully commit. Stick to chips, pizza, cheese, and decorated cup-cakes; anything beyond that will be lost on the crowd. You don't want people to be afraid of disturbing the spread, and grabby guests don't want dishes intended for visual appreciation anyway. They want a pretzel bowl they can go into palms open and leave fists full. Or just scrap it all and opt for a potluck. Let everybody else worry about it.

Games

There is usually a split vote on games at baby showers with each group residing on completely opposite ends of the spectrum. This is surprising since baby shower games are famous for being objectively god-awful, but there are still those among us who are willing to bust kneecaps if you don't whip out at least one. A game isn't going to kill anybody (at least, it shouldn't), and even if you aren't feeling it, you may discover their worth by watching others play. Confused and abrasive grand-mothers are usually a great place to fix one's atten-tion on, especially when their hearing aid batteries are dying. Here are a few suggestions that TodaysParent.com promises will be tolerated by just about anybody (but you're going to have to look past the names):

- **Rock 'n' Rattle:** Already a bad start. The web-site says this is a chance for guests to customize white onesies with cute and clever "rock and roll" verbiage. It sounds a little too cool for school, but don't put away the markers yet. Just drop the theme and have friends design the onesies however the hell they want. Your infant won't be caught dead in any of them, regardless.

- **Celebri-Baby:** Prepare pictures of celebrity offspring, and have people write down the ones they recognize. This idea sounds a little unexplored, and you can dress it up further. One of our friends took the Hollywood route with a twist by reciting out-to-lunch parenting quotes from famous celeb mamas. It was up to guests to guess who said what, and nobody kept score. Just listening to the disconnected and overentitled perspectives of ultra-rich women was reward enough for everyone.

- **And Bingo Was His/Her Name-O:** You know the drill. The grid is populated with common shower gifts (blankets, sleepers, diapers, etc.). Friends play as you open them. In a nutshell, it's a roundabout way for you to hold guests' attention while your "Christmas" comes early and has absolutely nothing to do with anyone's partialness to Bingo. To make things interesting for everyone, consider coughing up some prizes. Throw free items into the mix and people will submit themselves to just about anything.

A Baby Sprinkle/You've Got to be Kidding Me

Yes, we said "a baby sprinkle," and just reading it should make you want to slap yourself. It's one of those phrases you can barely bring yourself to repeat, because it feels like a trap set by a jerk to catch someone sounding like an idiot. Like the trap Starbucks laid when they named one of their tastiest cookies "Toffee Doodles." No self-respecting human being should ever be made to speak those words aloud; pointing and tapping on the display case like some sort of wingnut is a much more dignified way to place an order. Baby sprinkles, which are essentially multiple mini baby showers, are built on the idea that they're unnecessary, so at least they aren't afraid to be who they are. It's common knowledge among the mommy community that having more than one baby shower is a big no-no, and yet there are still those shameless few who will capitalize on the prenatal merriment over and over. And you know what? It makes sense. No questions, no guilt—just hand over the presents.

It's not so hot for everyone else. Another lame, reoccurring party—just what everyone needs. Baby sprinkles let women justify the second, third, or fourth shower by claiming it's been appropriately downgraded (*just a sprinkle this time, they swear!*). Well, if you can't help yourself from going back for shower seconds, at least have the decency to call it like it is and ditch the term "sprinkle." You're not fooling anyone. Just use the word "party" and call it a day!

Afterthoughts (Thank You Notes)

Love, honesty, respect, and thank you notes—that's how important these are to some women. The absence of penned gratitude following the giving of a gift can really stick in our craws. Is it because we are in constant pursuit of validation? Or is it because, by age thirty, most of us are irreversibly bitter and fated to take everything incredibly personally? That's a tough one, it truly is.

Some people, like Allison, can side with thank you notes (which is crazy because she has disastrous penmanship). Others hate them—or, to clarify, they hate the *impersonalized* versions. What is the point of spending the few minutes it takes to write a note if you don't take that extra second to acknowledge what the guest gave you and how it made you feel? But the real issue has nothing to do with how glorious or inglorious anyone is making these totems of appreciation; it's that notes have come to carry more weight than actual face-to-face thank-yous. We're sorry, but what's so great about a hard copy? How did human interaction get dethroned by a piece of paper that doesn't care who you are or how much you spent? It's like that old saying: if a tree feels thankful in the forest, but neglects to jot down just *how much*, was it really grateful in the first place?

On the other hand (and there is always another hand), some of us do have a knack for taking a thank you note and turning it into an up-to-date summary of an entire friendship, which is unequivocally lovely. In these cases, what you end up with is not just a card but a new addition to the mantlepiece (and a way to demonstrate to houseguests that you're amazing). Now that's something worth displaying and something that won't make it to the trash, *at least* until the next big move.

Don't get bent out of shape if your good intentions sit on your bedside table unsent. No one gets around to writing them until a few weeks after all the gift-giving, and by that point your motivation to undertake the tedium might forsake you. If you feel compelled to distribute, ask for help to get your little envelopes of amity out into the world. So, what if they're late? The people that matter will understand, and the people who don't understand don't deserve one anyway.

Thank God That's Over

Once the baby shower has wrapped, let it die. They come and go in a blink, and once it's all cleaned up and the handouts are packed away in your vehicle, you are ready to move on. Maternity is all about going full-speed ahead, from one milestone to the next, and there's not much time to stop and reflect on any of the hiccups anyway. Even if your shower (or sprinkles) is just one fail after another, you don't have time to give a rat's ass. You'll be too busy writing those pesky thank you notes.

MATERNITY PHOTO SHOOTS

Undeniable Photo Evidence of Your Decline into Motherhood

Buckle up. You're about to go on a roller-coaster ride of emotion via a series of dangerously intimate photos of yourself, your partner, and your belly (which for this shoot will be filling in for the part of "baby"). You may have noticed that most women can't get enough of themselves, and pregnancy doesn't slow the naval-gazing one bit. For years, self-fascination has driven moms to hallmark their expansion, beginning with the very early stages and continuing past the point where no one cares anymore. How long will it take before your love for the limelight leads you away from the bathroom mirror and into the big leagues i.e., the maternity photo shoot?

Before you get any ideas, let's get one thing straight. Pregnancy does something to women. It can, for lack of a better term, make them *totally* lame. Not permanently, but it is what it is. Luckily, this is a quality your maternity photo shoot will heavily rely on—the more embarrassing the stage, the richer the results. We're looking for tender moments, elevated by a kind of absurdity capable of providing both you and your friends a lifetime's worth of laughter. A perfectly executed maternity photo shoot by someone who "knows what they're doing" (*so* subjective) is a gift that just refuses to stop giving. Even when you unfollow it on Facebook.

You're Not a Professional/Send in the Professionals

Undoubtedly, you're no stranger to having your photo taken. Not because you're crazy-famous with paparazzi in constant pursuit (unless you are—look at you!), but because everybody these days is an active participant in the selfie movement, and the majority happen to be women. Just as Oprah Winfrey says "Here's what I know for sure," here's what *we* know: nothing is going to get in between a woman and her selfie game. Not a pregnancy, not a changing physical frame, and not even parenting, for that matter. Just look at Kim Kardashian. She took things to another level when she broke out a move mothers had only dared contemplate but never had the gall to do: she turned a family photo into a selfie by cropping out *her child*. Try following that performance.

Granted, by that time, North West was already of the external variety as opposed to the internal, but the point remains: women will always need to be the stars of their own life show. You're not going to slow your photo roll because of some kid, *especially* your own. This isn't to say you're planning to turn your maternity shoot into a series of head shots, but old habits die hard, even the selfie habit of a grown-ass woman.

With your photo-journaling obsession firmly in place, friends can expect a decrease in content value across all social media accounts. The maternity photo shoot pretty much follows the same trajectory:

Start with yoga pants.
Ensure feet are bare.
Pull up tank top.
Turn body to the side.
One hand on the belly.
One hand taking the selfie.
Initiate a wave of eye-rolls across Instagram.

Anyone can snap a picture, but only a professional can capture a moment. And you deserve a professional, as do those subjected to the subsequent barrage of photos. Only the pros will be able to take the magic invisible to the un-pregnant eye and translate it successfully to digital form. All the magical eyes meeting between partners, the magical positioning of the body and the magical semi-disrobing. Staged memories, on record, immortalized for eternity.

Choosing a Photographer

Use your eyes and look at anyone around you. Now, look at someone else. Now, look in the mirror. Chances are, every person you've just seen is an up-and-coming photographer. Two of the three will have business cards. One of the three has worked with someone outside of their immediate family. And none will have had any formal training. It's become impossible to not throw a stone in a crowd without hitting a photographer, but finding *the* photographer? That's a tough one.

Wanting the best and affording the best do not always go hand in hand. For example, Jillian wants a Land Rover Discovery, but she barely affords a Jeep Compass (it's . . . not the same). Allison wants a . . . well, Allison's doing pretty good. If a compromise must be made, you can pinch pennies without sacrificing the "spice" by selecting an individual with loose expertise and oodles of misplaced confidence. Someone with a flair for the hokey side of life and who can re-create the same dramatic tone that one gets from, say, a grown man in a cheap fedora. Someone who, based on the low bar we've just set and the prevalence of shutterbugs, we deduce you already know . . .

According to our calculations, half your graduating class is staking their claim in this field, assembling amateur "portfolios" (which, just so you know, is now a synonym for putting together an online album) and charging next to nothing. Facebook is rife with these characters, and they would really appreciate it if you threw them a bone. Honestly, whether you pay fifty or five hundred dollars, the whole event will be teeming with silliness—one minute you're pulling into the studio, and the next you have your stomach painted like a basketball, with your partner standing limply by in an oversized Chicago Bulls jersey. Don't fight the magnitude of the theatrics: you're only pregnant once (well, some of you), and each moment that passes is a moment that shouldn't be missed. Really—don't miss a thing. You're waddling through a comedic goldmine. Every flamboyant shot is a chance for you and your unborn to become a viral meme, and although a bad photographer increases your odds, you still need the right directives to clinch that status:

Popular Poses—Don't Ask Me Why

- **Looking down:** If you start by looking at the camera, then you need to take five until you can pull it together. When it comes to maternity photo shoots, moms must *always* look toward their abdominal protrusion in a blatant attempt to thwart the cryptic nature of the images. When you forget to stare at your belly, your audience may mistake a beautiful testament to life for the glamour shots of an extremely bloated woman. This is why a tractor-beam-like gaze down at your baby's temporary housing arrangements will eliminate any confusions and cue the appropriate "oohing" and "aww-ing."

- **All hands on the belly, partner at the back:** This is a classic. Your significant other stands behind you while both parents place their hands somewhere along the bottom of the belly, looking life-threateningly impassioned and ridiculous all at the same time. When done correctly, this image should provoke sentiments similar to those one might experience when scanning a public bathroom for a free stall and accidentally locking eyes with a stranger between the door and the doorframe.

- **Every hand on the belly, turned to the side:** This is the exact same pose, but the photographer will snap you and your partner from, that's right, the *side* (mind equals blown). Boobs and baby will look enormous. The dudes are going to dig this one.

- **Partner on knee, kissing belly:** This pose can create tension if held for too long. Your emotional vulnerability may falsely interpret the attention your partner is paying to the baby as attention that should be paid to you, causing you to crumble and sob. Crying is like hitting the reset button. You'll get a water break, a burst of encouragement from everyone in the room, and maybe a little back rub in the spirit of appeasement. Lean into your feelings. This is art, after all.
- **Hands placed in a heart shape on the belly:** Because nobody could possibly understand the love parents have for their unborn children, this hand position demonstrates just that in a way the "less blessed" can understand. Pictures like these leave Jillian wondering why no one makes heart shapes on *her* body. And when she eventually snaps out of her baby-fever dream, she's in the ice cream aisle of the grocery store, alone, wearing a sweater she swore she would get rid of months ago. Life.

Let's Get Original

Boring is so, well, boring. There aren't many surprises left to uncover in a standard maternity photo series, so bring as personalized a touch as possible. There really are no rules as to what will or won't fly, so while you're more than welcome to plug your own ideas or sample from those provided above, our suggestions below will take your shoot from zero to hero.

- **Involve a weapon or two:** You'll think we're being crass, but according to our North American search engines, nothing says "we're ready to welcome someone into our family" like holding a gun, so gather up your firearms (but please, only the appropriate ones) and start posing. Unfortunately, you can only hold two at a time, but don't let that hinder your creativty, and don't be afraid to point the weapon directly into the camera. Just for good measure.

- **Belly art:** This is a thing, and it's up to you to decide if it's a "do" or a "Holy shit . . . never." We bet having your stomach treated as a canvas would be relaxing, but what are women meant to do once it's all said and done? Stand there? Take one or two photos? What do you do with a hand-painted cycloptic eyeball (a popular choice for reasons we cannot even begin to imagine)? It's a lot of work for a photo that takes only seconds to capture, and watching it be wiped away has got to suck for the artistic mastermind behind it.

- However, if you are intrigued but hope for something with more substance, why not have that person paint your current anatomical makeup—to scale? If you're game, you can even request that the essential organ systems be added, squeezed in and around the free-hand doodle of your unborn. Graphic, but also a great way to brush up on what exactly is hiding behind all that skin and muscle.

- **Climb a tree:** Mix it up! Obeying gravity? How vanilla. You can do better than that—get outdoors. One of the best maternity shots floating around the web is of a mom in a tree. Juxtaposing unexpected themes like pregnancy and greenery is only one way to go; think of the buzz you'll create if you were to appear in an abandoned rowboat or sitting atop a deactivated cannon.

- **Involve props:** When you're standing in front of a cheap backdrop, blinded by an unprofessional lighting system, wondering "what next?," reach for the props to take things from zero to sixty. For example, Google "Leonardo DiCaprio and banana," and you'll find an otherwise average teen-dream poster that's set itself apart by incorporating a bed of fruit and some banana hands. Consider this the control to which all great prop-based photos should be measured. Save the blocks, chalkboards, and baby shoes for unadventurous norm-cores. Think outside the box, or involve a box (or maybe two?). Even a spare tire works. Don't believe us? It's already been done (see: the Internet).

- **Get out the boobs:** Nobody's "cans" are pregnant, so why are they always stealing the show? It's because people can't get enough of them. That's why it's so common to incorporate them, at one point or another, during these sessions. In many instances, you'll be chaperoning your own chest, but if you want to tap into your inner minx, you can always let your partner usurp the role of breast wrangler. If the swollen belly wasn't a big enough clue that the two of you are having sex, the flagrant manhandling should be a dead giveaway.

- **Both going topless:** Sure, maybe you've got your top off, but to crank the awkward dial to full blast, your significant other is going to have to get top-less, too. Now you can finally grant your social network full disclosure to how the top half of your sexual encounters might appear. But wait, do those people actually want to see their close friends pressed together in a nude embrace? We think you already know the answer. They wouldn't.

Snap! Snap! Snap!

That's a lot of priceless advice. If you can keep this chapter on hand for future reference, you'll be well on your way to collecting photographic material destined for festival entries and award consideration. Until then, your focus can rely on the fact that you are naturally captivating, without gimmicks or filters. You're pregnant, for god's sake! You're Mother Nature incarnate! Vogue! Vogue!

BUILDING A ~~NEST~~ NURSERY

You Are Still *Not an Interior Designer*

You've made it through the baby shower, you've managed to produce semi-appealing maternity photos, and now it's time for you to bang out the baby room. The nursery is where pregnant women can take everything they learned from assembling their childhood dollhouses and apply it to real life (if you are offended by our assumption that you played with dolls, first ask yourself why, and then relax). As youngsters, *we* were doll people. Allison had the whole upstairs of her shed converted into every girl's dream, a sprawling network of mini-mansions and Fold 'n' Fun Houses we called "Barbie World." Jillian had a handmade multiplex, which looked a little different than Allison's setup. Please, contain your jealousy, because in saying "handmade," she's referring to *her* own hands, which meant creating however many storied homes with her father's speakers and fashioning furniture from empty toilet paper rolls and paper plates. Her "Barbs," as she called them, had more than enough bedrooms, sunrooms, guest rooms, and garages for the caravan and corvette, and, yes, there was even a nursery—where else would the Quints sleep?

It's unlikely you're planning rooms around five infants as we once did, but there's definitely at least *one* you need to consider. Most women designate a single room in their home to "baby-fy"—in fortunate or unfortunate ways. The choice is yours. Although friends may not be involved in the actual execution of the nursery, you may need them to serve as fully animated and articulated sounding boards. You will bulldoze besties with endless streams of prospective concepts and designs. You will have family and friends running their eyes over various types of nurseries, themed and un-themed, as well as individual necessities big and small, i.e., cribs, changing tables, window treatments, and paint colors. Things are ostentatious from the get-go (Deluxe Paint Mixing in "Soft Gooseberry," anyone?), and don't forget to pepper the walls with pink or blue anchors so visitors know how hip to the sailing and/or ocean scene you plan to pretend to be.

If it sounds exhausting, that's because it will be—for you. For your gal pals? At its worst, they'll be halfway irritated, and that's only if the minutia is lost on them. To be an effective contributor, all anyone needs is the ability to offer up an opinion *when asked for one*. There will be conversations where outside interest is sincere and others in the name of feelings and manners. Whatever the case, friends are there to keep you picking away at the process and to make sure you avoid getting, and staying, stuck. There are no rewards for tormenting yourself with particulars or being stifled by the inherently female predisposition to overthink *everything*. If so, our homes would be 90 percent trophies (we'll give that remaining 10 percent to unrequited sexual advances).

Why All the Fuss

Looking at all the possibilities when designing a nursery makes those who are not in the maternal way, in a word, grateful. Grateful that they aren't the ones who are suddenly expected to become a tasteful and effective interior decorator. There are all sorts of ways you can screw this one up, even if you're trying your damnedest not to. But why is everyone so adamant to get it so right in the first place? So much fuss and muss. If you ask us (which, sadly, not enough people do), women who work toward nursery perfection are motivated partly by their own personal satisfaction and largely by their quest for houseguest approval (especially from those with kids of their own). The baby doesn't care about his or her amenities. Maybe we have too much momentum when it comes to family prep. We stray from the essentials because we can't help ourselves. Just ask the multiple ribbon-bound storage solutions in Allison's daughter's bedroom that, although practical in theory, have remained empty since their installation, or the wire birdcage in Jillian's living room that she impulsively bought to fill with books she wants people to think she's read. But enough about us. Let's look at the most important concerns you should keep in mind when putting this space together.

- **Lighting:** Not too bright. Those eyeballs are fresh, and the number of times they have opened and closed may still be in the double digits. The answer is probably as simple as a dimmer switch and a set of dark/thick curtains. Duh.
- **Color:** The interiors of life rafts are blue to promote calmness. Okay, but it's going to take a lot more than a periwinkle hue to stave off panic in abandoned passengers. The point is, there is science in color. Stay away from hot or harsh shades. You don't want a neon pink room screaming into your baby's peepers. Or maybe you do; bring on the Jazzberry Jam.
- **Temperature:** Don't freeze the baby. Don't cook the baby. Your baby is a person, and you know a

bit about that, so aim for temperatures you have found pleasant in the past. If it's summer, a fan, AC, or dehumidifier may be required to get the air just right, and sometimes all three. Sure, these electronic eyesores will stick out like sore thumbs within the sugary-sweet four walls of your baby's new abode, but sometimes it's substance before style. Or hideous devices over heat rash.

- **Texture:** Keep things soft; plush, even. No chain-mail. No studs.

- **Content:** When was the last time you ever saw a baby of changing station age spending time at a desk? Unless you're building a movie set for the sixth installment of the Baby Geniuses franchise, it doesn't make sense. Don't overshoot your kids' capabilities. That hobby horse in your two-week-old's room isn't going to ride itself, and unless your son or daughter is possessed, neither will he or she. Stick to a crib, rocking chair, and stocked changing table. You might want to consider a Diaper Genie, too. Never underestimate the power of the genie, especially the one that grants the wish of unpolluted air.

And the rest is just superfluous accenting. The bric-a-brac that makes mommy feel accomplished, not baby.

We're not saying there isn't value in frills and extra touches. They *can* make things fun, and let's be honest: moms and fun have a strained relationship in need of serious attention. Putting together a nursery could be your chance to reconnect with "a good time" (a relative term, that's for sure), and you might as well incorporate your loved ones while you're at it. And they *will* help. Who wouldn't jump at the chance to channel *Designing Women*, particularly when only one of you will be footing the bill (can you guess who it won't be)?

Balls Deep into Basics

Color is huge, and we are, at this moment, sending you however many influential vibes it's going to take for you to go with something muted and subtle (remember, hot and harsh: *bad*). You want something that won't need a complete overhaul as the baby grows and that is also gender neutral; ultrasounds *have* been wrong in the past. Committing to a grossly stereotypical boy or girl theme welcomes the chance that this room will either come with an expiration date, or just be tacky. White water, Sweet Innocence, Feather, and Silver Half Dollar are all gray paints that appear completely interchangeable to the un-invested eye, so let your besties tap out until you've narrowed it down to your top three contenders. In the end, it will be up to you to decide which will look best on your chevron-patterned wall.

Once you've made those decisions, it's time to furnish the little miracle's surroundings. When, you will ask yourself, did it become so hard to choose a dresser? Or a crib? Or a changing table whose sole purpose is to provide a permanent de-shitting area? What is it about any of these objects that warrants such thorough deliberation? The baby doesn't care about light or dark stains; the baby *makes* stains. You know this, you just keep forgetting to care.

The greatest threat to realizing your cutesy-comfy-cohesive vision will be your access to the Internet (cue evil music). Just as Facebook should have a breathalyzer to avoid drunk status updates and rage messaging, Pinterest should be running urine tests to restrain pregnant women. Scrolling through other peoples' good ideas is addictive, and if you let too many of them creep into your assembly process, you will overdose. Don't compromise the traditional simplicity of a soft and serene nursery by over-committing and over-ornamenting.

The Bad, the Bad, and the Ugly

It's not unheard of for women to pull from Beatrix Potter while modeling their baby rooms. Makes sense, who wouldn't want to spend time inside a children's book full of talking animals? We do ask that you please not get too overwrought by the watercolor, ribbons, and Jemima Puddleduck-ness of it all. Coco Chanel once said, "Before leaving the house, a lady should look in the mirror and remove one accessory." This is a transferable skill. Come back to this mantra when you're up to your ears in framed versions of the alphabet and Disney character decals. Always take a step back and remove one (or more) items. You want your baby to feel at ease, not have a seizure.

Overstating the Obvious

There is a nursery bedding set on eBay that is "Every Shade of Purple/*Zootopia*"-themed, and it has got to be one of the worst things in the world. It's a muddle of mismatched prints and fabrics, and the photo used by the seller to lure consumers showcases a truly gruesome scene where a blank slate of a room once stood. Still, many women long for a menagerie-styled area in which to lay their child. Animals are fun, but keep the details to a dull roar. The word *safari* doesn't need to be splashed across the blanket, the wall, and the mobile. People aren't idiots. They only need to see one zebra to figure out what direction you decided to go in.

Let Less Be Less, Not More

Pinks and creams are lovely, as are ruffles and bows, and we all know how timeless Christopher Robin's furry friends are, but it is possible to have too much of a good thing. It's possible to have too much of a bad thing, so if your nursery starts looking like something a strung out Strawberry Shortcake would put together, you need to stop what you're doing. You don't need more accents; you need restraint before your baby's room becomes overshadowed by an even more glaring theme: "unnecessary."

How to Raise an Asshole

While googling "pretentious nurseries" we came across the Shangri-La of kids' rooms. The bed was built like a castle, towers and all, and it had two evacuation slides on either end just long enough to give brats time to yell "Fuck Youuuuu" at all their less fortunate friends as they awake from their overprivileged rest and make their way to the ground. If you've ever wondered how to raise an asshole, this might be a great place to start. Of course, kids *want* a mini-kingdom and slides spilling off their bunk beds, but they shouldn't actually *get* them. When children make lavish demands, you are meant to laugh, hand them a spoon (wooden, not silver), and shove them outside to humble themselves with some good, old-fashioned dirt play. Indulging them now means facing the danger of a morbidly obese ego later.

Nesting

But enough with the don'ts and more don'ts. There is apparently a method to your madness—well, not a "method" per se, but at least an explanation. Moms and baby books alike will tell you that the reason you've been spending an inordinate amount of time obsessing over which wall decal to center above the cradle is because you're "nesting." Nesting is sort of like an offshoot of Mom Brain where you take a shining to housework and turn into Martha Stewart, if Martha Stewart had a bun in the oven (Wait, is *that* Martha's secret? Has she been pregnant for *forty* years?).

The term was lifted from our friends in the animal kingdom. Birds (obviously). Dogs. Cats. They all prepare for their broods by nesting. It's both fascinating and confounding to watch a pregnant lady figuring out how to rearrange her house when she can't climb, over-reach, or lift anything over two pounds. Take Allison, for example, a clean-and-organized-isolate-type who, whenever she invites Jillian over, is known to offer up water, only to then wash and put the glass back into the cupboard before a second sip can be taken. For other moms-to-be, this time is a great opportunity to suss out who stands where on your friend totem pole. Researchers have found that during this period, you'll only want to surround yourself with those most trusted (who can help you with a nesting chore, or two). If that's the case, Jillian's sister must trust her siblings *a lot*—they had to wipe down baseboards, blinds, and bannisters before their nephew arrived. The things you do for family. At least they made the cut?

Saying It's Perfect

It's all about keeping yourself on an appropriately sized leash through this time. Whatever the final decisions are, they will be, first and foremost, yours (and so will the blame). Be open to input during the design stages, because there isn't much point for criticisms when the paint has dried and the life-size wooden stork is secured against the wall. Landslide victory or not, the same golden rule of friendship applies: if you're happy, then they're happy, too (but we can't guarantee anyone's impressed).

THE BIRTH PLAN

Your Pièce de Résistance

It's up to you to call the shots when it comes to how you will care for yourself and your unborn child throughout a pregnancy. Women are rarely interested in people looming over their shoulders, telling them when to pop their prenatal vitamins or what times of the day are best to sneak in a few sets of Kegels. Well, the fact is mothers of the mom-to-be and mothers-in-law *have* been known to loom, and loom they will. For the most part, though, you should be able to waddle around to the beat of your own drum until the labor pains start. Picture it: you're doubled over, writhing in pain after your water breaks like a rogue wave—a rogue wave armed with a six-to-ten-pound renegade getting ready to "hang ten" as it surfs down the vaginal canal. It's tough keeping things from spiraling out of control. This is the point where, even if you are "keeping it real," your unborn child is going to be "keeping it real-er." Planning ahead can somewhat anchor the chaos. In hopes of salvaging their sanity, women jot down a list of pre-established conditions of delivery—and to make sure nobody will mistake the intent of the document, they call it a "birth plan."

If you recognize this phrase, then we'll assume you already have a firm grip on the concept. However straightforward it may seem, let us assure you that a birth plan can be anything but. This is a facet of pregnancy in which you see record variation. There is no "one size fits all," no Sisterhood of the Traveling Birth Plan, and that's what makes it so damn complicated. The more society advances and medicine allows women to birth on their own terms, the more elaborate these rosters become. Not that elaborate is bad; not that women shouldn't be able to choose how they bring their spawn into their lives. But if pregnant women were rock stars (and let's face it, they kind of are), the riders are starting to get a little over the top.

The birth plan is about making choices. Ever since we weren't allowed to choose *anything*, we've become obsessed with choosing *everything*. We only ever really know what we want after someone tells us what we cannot have. It's an awful, awful character trait, but since us gals have been granted almost total antenatal freedom, no one seems afraid to exploit the hell out of it. And once you realize that a birth plan is essentially just a contract stating that you, in a broad sense, "get your own way," you will be searching for the nearest sign-up sheet.

What is a Birth Plan?

A birth plan is like a very formal list of instructions that a woman will give her midwife, her doula, or her doctor, which insists upon an ideal delivery. That is, *your* ideal delivery, in extremely duteous detail. We're talking specifics of specifics here. Don't get shy when it comes to communicating personal preferences to those handling your labor. Everyone must be on the same page, which is hard to do when the page is of the literal rather than figurative sense. Plus, it isn't just *page*, it's pag-*es*. Although many of your wishes are no doubt reasonable, some women tread effortlessly into diva—or worse, crazy—territory.

We have heard of one such birth plan in which the woman had requested her husband be permitted to whisper words of encouragement into/at her vagina throughout the big day. That poor husband. His wife basically asked him to play a game of pass the whisper with her crotch and her asshole, and he *agreed*. Now we appreciate the inadvertent bawdiness of this couple, but clearly these are two people who have completely lost touch with reality, and frankly we are shocked they were at a clinic at all and not at home, getting tangled up in some sort of birthing swing. If that's not the most seminal case of the power of pregnancy, we don't know what is.

When to Write Up Your Plan

It doesn't matter how avid a reader you believe yourself to be; you've probably read more in the last five or six months than you have the last few years. And even though it's all been about the same subject, you've never tired of it, and now the time has finally come to share what you've learned. Getting an early start is smart. If you're going to have a tailor-made labor, you need to give the specialists enough notice. They're only doctors, remember, not mind readers. When a solid projection of the due date is established, go ahead and open a Word document: it's time to consolidate your deepest and darkest demands. But before you start penning your masterpiece, remember the value of flexibility, because these are the kinds of plans you can depend on to change. The chances of your birth plan being carried out to your exact specifications are about the same as your vag's and anus's chances of remaining next-door neighbors post-birth: not good.

How to Write Up Your Plan

Trying to churn out one of these freehand is like trying to clean a messy room with no organizational spaces or tools. Grab a template off the Internet to act as a spring-board to your final draft. Something akin to those "About Me" surveys we all used to fill out in elementary school ("My favorite color is _____"; "After school I like to play _____") but for women ("When I have my baby I want the lights _____"; "Ideally, I want my baby to emerge from my _____"). To avoid disappointment, keep it short, simple, and, above all, doable. This is meant to be a list, not a manuscript, and whoever is responsible for its execution won't make much headway if they have to rifle through reams of paper to follow along.

Manuscript or not, rewrites and revisions are always a good idea. Make first, second, and third drafts, and a stupid amount of copies. You don't need to rain these down the staircase of your old high school like "the coolest party ever" flyers, but the more people in the know, the better. That's one for the nurse, the practitioner, your partner, your dog, your mailman, and, of course, one special copy just for you.

Even with a template, it's hard to know where to begin. Though the details are anyone's guess, the skeleton remains consistent. Here are a few popular sub-sections found in birth plans (for reasons that fall far beyond our comprehension).

Getting Ready

- **Music:** some playlists are made to work out to, some are made to get busy to, but this will be made to have a baby to. What songs are going to put you in the mood to be a master-pusher? Will you have one steady theme across the board, i.e., rock anthems or jungle ambient? Or will you try to follow the progression of labor, starting off with some slow jams before moving into something frenzied frenzied like "Flight of the Bumblebee," ending with a triumphant chorus (maybe the score that plays as the helicopter first approaches Jurassic Park)? Whatever your musical tastes, here are a couple of nominees for your theoretical playlist.
  - *Don't Cry Out Loud*: This would be a neat song to push, or feel weird, to.
  - *My Ding-a-ling*: This should be considered the standard go-to for whenever a boy is born, for obvious reasons. Having a girl? Opt for something with a lilt, like *There's a Place in France*. Sure, the words don't really apply, but it's more about that melody, you know, the one that cartoon characters use to hypnotize snakes. Your body may not be as easy to exit as a basket,

but why not give it a go and see if it can charm your baby's way out as well?

- *My Humps*: A strong competitor for worst song in existence, "My Humps" may finally find its place in the world inside the walls of the delivery room. Aren't you in possession of the biggest and loveliest "lady lump" of them all? The hump to end all humps? What else are we supposed to do with this song? Seriously, Fergie, we're asking.

- The song that plays as the Wicked Witch of the West first appears in Dorothy's window during the tornado. You know it: "*Do do do do do do do, do do do do do do do, dooooooooooooo.*" This one isn't for you; it's for your midwife, doula, or doctor to play on their cellular devices as they watch your car pull into the parking lot.

- **Lighting:** Well, you're going to need at least one light on, that's for sure. We're not experts, but delivering in the dark cannot be beneficial for anyone. One wrong move and what was meant to be a standard delivery turns into an emergency extraction of a pair of forceps from one very startled ass. So, once you've decided yes, indeed lights on *is* best, we're not sure what other decisions need to be made here. Are there births being held by candlelight? The woman with the vagina-whispering husband would probably be game for that.

The Main Event

- **Pushing:** It's said that people with IBS are pro pushers—so, they're basically saying labor is like trying to take the hugest shit of your life, with more crowd-pleasing results. You have to push when you go through contractions. Push like you're trying to blow your legs off, and if that doesn't sound helpful, you should know that there are techniques proven to speed things along. Techniques based on timing and movement that are probably worth looking into since there's a good chance you'll be at this for hours. Almost everyone is.

- **Positions:** Throughout the intensity of labor, it's going to be hard for you to not give into your body's cues and contort into a reluctant human pretzel. Rest assured there are ways for you to find "comfort," or at least find comfort in your discomfort. Think of all the different sex positions you and your friends have discussed over the years, or the ones you picked up during bikini waxing sessions. Getting through labor may mean having to settle into almost all of them a few times over. On all fours is a popular one, or, as we like to call it, "Anal Bleaching Stance." There is also the wide-based squat, a.k.a. "where dignity goes to die." You know what they say about birthing positions: the more the merrier, and maybe with enough twists and turns of your body, your little one will finally come loose.

- **Using a mirror:** What are people thinking with this mirror business? We can't be the only women who can barely bring ourselves to glimpse *that* area on a good day, let alone the day when it's being put through the ringer. If you're up to the challenge, you may want to test yourself before you get an eyeful of cooch. YouTube is a great place to do this. There are thousands of channels featuring clips that will shed some light on what lies ahead. So much light, in fact, that you may have to turn away. You may have seen one such video. A woman's family appears to be spending some wholesome, quality time at a really shitty beach when, suddenly, you hear a sound, the kind Little Foot's mother would have made if her death scene in *The Land Before Time* had used more realistic audio. The camera then pans to a woman, naked, in a full-on squat, with a baby about to drop onto a river bend (at least we assume it was a baby; at that stage they all look like picnic hams). At about forty-five seconds in, we had to call it a day. Everyone took sex-ed in middle school so we know how that story ends, but the live-action movie version is . . . simian and absolutely horrifying. Maybe you're into that; maybe you'd find it heartening. Maybe it gives you the boost you need to carry you right on through to the end. Mirror or no mirror, at least your friends will never have to gaze into that reflection with you, if ever. Shivers.

- **Video recording:** Let's get back to filming. Videotaping is about capturing ~~a series of box shots~~ the essence of the occasion. We're guessing you have chosen to birth far away from bodies of water, but just because the setting of your delivery may not be as "wild" as the YouTube woman's doesn't mean there won't be just as much *Naked and Afraid*. Not sure how many women would consent to this, but one thing we know for certain— Allison was *not* one of them. That doesn't mean tape wasn't rolling at some point. During midcontraction and without her knowledge (but not necessarily against her will), her husband managed to seize some "live moments" from inside the waiting room. In a brief thirty-second clip, she is shown lumbering around like a "drunken sloth" (her words) and gripping onto metal chairs as if she were Bruce Banner steadying himself for the Hulk's resurgence. It's the sort of mini-movie that only surfaces for the most private of screenings, but it remains one of Allison's favorites because, as it turns out, her feral self is a physical comedy genius and an unlikely source of joy.

Then there is Jillian, who, without a first-hand encounter to call her own, must put herself in her friend's stirrups to truly appreciate the potential horrors of video-ed delivery. She always pictures the same scenario: she's herself, but she's also Regan McNeil from *The Exorcist*. She's strapped to a hospital bed, in that terrible nightgown, with grotesque makeup, wheezing like she's mistaken the "Ghost Pepper Wing Sauce" over traditional "Hot" (*again*). As her partner pans the camera across the room and asks oh-so-innocently how she's feeling, she looks straight through the lens and hisses, *"Your mother sucks cocks in hell!"* That would be Jillian—the devil incarnate.

Here's the rub: if you want to make a flick, then you are going to make a flick, and no matter what happens there is no way it could ever be as frightening as the scene described above. Videos are just for mom and dad anyway; they're intensely intimate and not really something to be shared with family and friends. Because, yes, that *is* too much to ask.

- **Company kept:** Who holds the backstage passes? It is suggested that your birth plan outline when you would and would not like your supporting partner(s) to stay with you for certain procedures, conversations, etc. But can you be expected to adhere to these decisions when you're actually in those moments? For example, say your partner is, in an (un)foreseen turn of events, driving you up the wall, and you need a break for a few minutes. Will the doctor or midwife defer to the birth plan and veto your request because you had stated, in writing, that you wanted him or her by your side? We doubt it. Just more stipulations that everyone could have done without, making it a section of the birth plan you may want to skip altogether.
- **Eating and drinking during labor:** The best you can expect is Jell-O and popsicles. It's the "you just had your wisdom teeth or tonsils out" diet, but instead of getting sufficiently gassed and handing all the real work over to the professionals,

you're going to have to perform this procedure practically alone, relying on your own endurance and temporary insanity. Having played a few sports in our time, we can't recall any of our coaches or teammates ever pushing us to get more "Jell-O" or other refrigerated treats into our systems for the necessary refuel at half-time. You're being asked to run a marathon here, but there's been a ban placed on the protein shakes and power bars you desperately need. Damn; those Cool Mint Chocolate CLIF BARs were probably on sale, too.

- **Pain relief:** If you ask Jillian, the best way to go through labor would be to have someone knock her out cold during the first contraction (preferably with a swift punch to the face), only to be roused once everything was over and done with. She wants it to be like Christmas: you go to sleep, somebody takes care of the things that need taking care of, and you wake up with presents all laid out for you. But childbirth isn't like Christmas, apart from the fact that they start with the same consonant, and we still live in a time when delivering an invited smack to a pregnant woman is taboo. Therefore, if she were to ever give birth, she would need to rely on the more conventional methods of pain relief—the epidural.

Now, we all know about epidurals, but we're not sure what they *are* or at least what they do on a molecular level. We've heard it can put an end to suffering, and maybe that's all women really need to know when in dire straights. Women like Allison. For her, this was a chance to take pretty hard narcotics without abandoning any hard-earned moral integrity. Allison was a kid who, even into our teens, was strongly against drug use, something that was never more apparent than when you caught her attempting to wrangle a cigarette. She was the "Just Say No" campaign personified, and whenever someone would suggest we "live a little," she would be the first to counter, "No, we really shouldn't." But pain changes you, especially labor pains, and by her second centimeter of dilation she was begging the nurses for morphine. What's more amazing is how little time it took between that initial hit and her standing in the shower, naked and vomiting all over herself because *someone* couldn't handle her opiates. Did we mention that her husband and doctors all bore witness to this mess?

Despite beautiful experiences like Allison's, there are those who bypass the meds completely. Whether you are a masochist, you want to "go big or go home," or you just have "something to prove," rest assured that no one is going to force you to numb your pain in ways you're not comfortable with. There are non-chemical options to calm your nerves and physical distress. For example, breathing exercises are bigger than ever right now. They are meant to target the agony, but they're also massively irritating, which might be all the distraction you need. We're sure every woman would rather feel annoyed than like their bodies were being halved. If all the controlled inhaling and exhaling isn't working for you, try coaxing a relaxed state with some light petting. This is the one day when you will get a massage out of just about anyone, so cash in those chips over and over and over.

After Party

- **Cutting the cord:** Though we have met many women (and many more men) whose umbilical cords are still fiercely intact even into their thirties and forties, the majority of us have them cut fresh after the birth. It's a snip that has become meaningful, often performed by a loved one—why, we cannot be sure. Maybe it's the adult version of having your mom wipe your bum as a kid, a gross demonstration of care. Or maybe it's just the new mom's way of throwing someone a bone so they can say they did something that day, too (while she rolls her eyes at them in the background).

- **Placenta:** Good grief, people and their placentas. You'd think these women were alchemists transmuting after-birth to gold. Although it has gotten a lot of good press over the last few decades with claims to lower the risk of postpartum depression, restore hormonal balance, and act as a great meat substitute for those sick of plain old beef burritos or chicken salad sandwiches, the fact remains that a placenta is a part of a person's body. A part that we have apparently developed a taste for. No longer does it have to be in the middle of the Andes Mountains in 1972 for people to be interested in their own remains—all the cool moms are chowing down voluntarily; and the hipper they are, the more inventive they get. Placenta stew, placenta pâté, placenta pills. There are so many methods of preparation, but does a woman's chosen path of ingestion make the thought any less unpleasant? If someone were to say to you after an appendectomy "... and then I ate it," you would raise an eyebrow, maybe two. But if their clarifying statement was something like "Well, I *encapsulated* it first," or "Don't worry, I blended it into a smoothie, would it really make all the difference? Or *any*? No matter the technique, the result is the same: something that clearly wanted out of your system being is stuffed back in. They might as well stock the maternity ward with Styrofoam take-out containers, because all we can imagine are these women, newly born babies in one arm and placenta in the other, asking their obstetricians if they can get theirs "to go." And yes, some will argue for the "naturalness" of it by noting that animals do this all the time, our beloved domesticated dogs included, but *we* would argue that many of those same canines have also been known to eat their own feces, so perhaps someone should re-examine that measure for diet standards.

To tell the truth, we're playing devil's advocate here; we aren't really against any of this. Not against the women participating in human placentophagy and not against exploring its benefits. But it *does* make us slightly uneasy, like that squirmy feeling you get whenever you're driving and you spot *very* grown men and women crammed in the backseat of another adult's vehicle (you don't know why it feels wrong, but it sure *does*). If you do end up taking the plunge by running yours through your body once more for good luck, then we offer our power to you. Just don't post any photos on Facebook. *Just don't post any photos on Facebook.*

- **Circumcision:** So, you're Jewish. If you're not, then we're not sure why this could possibly make its way into your birth plan. It's a religious practice, not a sanitary one. Don't let them get you on that. How many uncircumcised men do you know who have had compromised health issues, who became severely ill, or who died because they still had their foreskin? If we're going to delve into issues of cleanliness, these dudes should try having a vagina, for Christ's sake. Let the little guys get comfortable in their own skin before you let someone hack it off. Besides, introducing a baby to plastic surgery at the age of ten minutes cannot be good for self-confidence in the long run.

What Now?

You should have your birth plan looked over by someone who knows what they're talking about—not just you and whoever else is willing to keep a straight face for the twenty-minutes-too-many it takes to read through to the end. Feedback is important if you want to stay practical. Going into a birth expecting, for example, a water delivery with nature sounds playing in the background while your partner reads French Renaissance poetry aloud is setting yourself up for disappointment. Not just because that's clearly deluded, but also because births, by nature, love to go off script. In the end, you will likely have to give up a few of your ideals (in the previous case, we would drop the waxing poetic fool, for good). And, appreciate what goes your way. Actually, appreciate everything—that's a good one.

SECTION 4
THE AFTER-BIRTH

THIS IS BABY WHAT'S-HIS/HER-FACE

What's the Word for When Something Is Both Exciting and "Holy Fuck?"

Not everyone is going to have kids, and not everyone is going to *want* to have kids, but it doesn't mean women can't and don't swell with joy whenever someone dear to them becomes a mother. If you were to peel back all the snark, the sarcasm, and the negative bias, you'd find that every decent woman is pretty much built on the same well-intentioned foundation: we just want each other to be happy.

With that in mind, let's switch gears for a moment, set the jokes aside, and give women in general the credit they deserve. Let's hear it for you (having just birthed a little human). It takes a lot of blood, sweat, tears, and numerous other unspeakable bodily fluids to get this far. And to say that child production is an "accomplishment" would be an understatement bordering on insult. Sure, we all have accomplishments that carry personal significance and make us proud. This book, for instance, or that time Jillian was able to get a high-end skin care company to send her a full bottle of facial serum to "replace" the one she lied about buying in the first place. And although everyone she talks to is consistently impressed with her ability to swindle the multimillion-dollar beauty industry, the birth of a child, like the one Allison managed to squeeze out, is in a league of its own. Not a *better* league, we should make it clear, just a very different one. A revelatory league with a hefty entry fee and one life-changing payoff—but we don't have to tell you that. *You*, however, do have to tell everyone.

A typical birth announcement is a photo with basic stats attached, i.e., name, weight, height, date, time of birth, and parents' names (you've got your wagon hitched tightly to this little star, haven't you). They're like delightful varieties of those old "Wanted" posters you see in Spaghetti Westerns, and just like the posters that inspired them, their charm can be short-lived, and sometimes even destroyed.

Depending on Mom and Dad, details included in a birth announcement can end up extending way beyond what any recipient needs to know. Like when you confirm that your baby *does* have all his or her extremities. Yes, that is unbeatable, and *of course* we want them accounted for, but that's just business as usual, isn't it? As in, it's "assumed unless otherwise stated," the same way we would assume your baby was also born with one of those heads we so often see atop of people these days, along with two arms and two legs to match. And although we appreciate that not all of us are necessarily put together in the same way, the announcement might not be the best place to discuss your baby's articulated body dynamics.

Aside from that, say what you will, and we mean that, because no one is going to fault you for going overboard on the announcement no matter how redundant the info. It's only natural to want to show what can be produced when you go almost a whole year without downing a tequila shot or waking up in a bed of empty Rock Star Vodkas (now there's an accomplishment worthy of some recognition). Nobody dared call Sarabi an "attention whore" when she had Rafiki thrust Simba into the air above the entire animal kingdom in what was possibly the most elaborate birth announcement ever (only to be later re-created and quite frankly *ruined* by Michael Jackson with his son Blanket in a terrifying ordeal that taught us Disney movies do *not* translate well in real life).

So, as long as you're not dangling your infant off a cliff in the middle of the African Sahara or over a balcony in Berlin, your birth announcement will be well received, and it will mean, your gloating has found a suitable *and* bearable context. Finally!

Some People Are Allergic to Well-Wishing

Allow us to partake in one of our favorite pastimes—shaking things up with a cold dose of reality. As you know, we're not operating under the diplomacy of a fictional lion's pride, but everyone has an "Uncle Scar" in their lives—somone who feels the need to chime in with snide remarks and who is physically unable to let you merry-make in your well-deserved glory. This will rub you and your friends in the most wrong of ways. Don't let them rain on your baby parade. Cut these people down and out of your life immediately. It's one thing to make fun of a woman's two-bit maternity photos, but ripping her proclamation of procreating a "new one" is a sign of some seriously depraved character. There is no room for haters from here on out, because, as sad as it is, adulthood isn't really bursting with opportunities to shine. It's characteristically fraught with successive exercises in personal disappointment, lost love, disillusionment, and having an all-around tendency of being a drag. Soak up the sunny moments, and your son's or daughter's birth is probably going to be one of your all-time sunniest. Let the baby bliss reign for as long as it can.

The Misadventures of Visiting Hours

Speaking of baby, let the face-to-face introductions commence. After hearing about him/her (incessantly) for the past year, friends finally get to size up what all the fuss is about. This interaction, however dazzling, can be awkward to navigate—and that's just among the adults. How do guests know when the visit is over—when you're too tired or when a welcome has been overstayed? How do they know what questions to ask now and what can wait until later? How do they know not to show up empty handed?

Jillian popped in to visit Allison after she had just given birth to her daughter, and upon her arrival Allison announced (in the most classic Allison way): "Don't say anything. I look like shit." The learned response here, as a concrete rule within the girl code, is a rebuttal without hesitation—only this time she wasn't wrong. Allison resembled one of those "things" your dog brings in from outside that makes you repeat over and over, in horror: "What is that? *What is that?*" So, while Jillian would usually refute her friend's self-deprecation, it was clear that any effort to contradict her this time was going to end in some form of violence (likely of the "slappy" sort). There's a valuable lesson here: although a positive assessment is great in clumsy situations, never underestimate the value in one's ability to read the room.

A few years later, after Allison was long discharged, Jillian and her family made an appearance at that very same hospital to visit her sister and her new nephew, and all she brought was a coffee—for herself. It didn't occur to her to bring anything else, not a balloon, not a card, and not even the words, "I'm stopping at Tim Hortons, did you want anything?" This was what she calls a "rookie mistake" and what Allison calls "very Jillian." A list really should be made accessible to all future maternity ward visitors outlining encouraged visitor etiquette to prevent similar faux pas.

It wouldn't hurt to clear up the confusion around who customarily receives the gifts. Are guests buying for baby from now on, or does the new mom have a couple things on her wish list, too? What do babies even want? Is it too soon for a rattle or a teething toy? The best answer we have is simply "ask"; another safe bet for those comfortable winging it is food.

Moms have worked up an appetite to no one's surprise. They say you can never go wrong with food, and no one in the history of childbirth has ever turned away a snack. Chocolate, whatever "bonbons" are, a casserole, coleslaw, those triangle sandwiches that Norm MacDonald is always after (and that always seem to be either tuna or egg), etc.—these are acceptable under the nonexistent screening process of the voracious new mother. You lucky dog. Before you know it, you'll be swimming in a sea of free and mismatched nibbles fit for a wake—which may sound morbid but is actually quite fitting since there is one loss in this equation worthy of a catered good-bye: your sacrificial vagina.

Tipping Our Hats to the Hoo-Hah (A Momentary/ Honorary Deviation)

With the massively objective gain of a baby comes this devastating cost. It's never easy to say goodbye to an old friend, especially one you grew up with. We're sure you both have been through a lot together, but the time has come to move onto the next stage of your co-existence. A somewhat "roomier" stage, and, much to your former self's dismay, a stage less frequented by your partner (for now). Women everywhere sympathize with you both (you and your vag, not you and your bae). If you listen ever so carefully, you can actually hear your snatch's swan song following you wherever you go—a hollow, resonant sound like the one made when blowing across the top of a bottle, except that's just the breeze blowing past your newly gutted undercarriage.

Because of this sexual handover—boobs become food, crotch becomes that cave from *The Descent*—you'll have to look to the secondhand sexual escapades of your gal pals to get your fill of heated moments (until you're able to start participating in your own again). And if they're also in a slump, no big deal—nothing brings friends together like commiserating over the thick layer of dust that's collecting on everyone's sex lives.

Wash Your Hands

The tables have turned. Five months ago, everyone thought *you* were the gross one, farting out of turn and sweating like a pig. Now, friends are the huge, derelict mess. Their hair is greasier than ever, their hands look like two fleshy bacterial breeding grounds, and you're convinced they're carrying hepatitis A through C. Just a bunch of hygienic disasters, turning you and your baby way off.

Your paranoia is well-placed. Now that you're a primary caregiver to someone with the immune system of a ninety-nine-year-old taking their last breath, everyone should educate themselves on external sterilization. In fact, getting clean and staying clean shouldn't be too much to ask; hopefully many adults are already doing this as part of their everyday routines. However, this level of commitment can mean a lot of upkeep. These aren't your typical standards of cleanliness, these are strict regulations built upon a foundation of new mothers' neurosis. So, if gals and guys want to hang out, they need to de-grime (meaning sponge baths are off the table, where they should have been all along).

The Main Attraction

Meeting a baby for the first time is one of the most awkward introductions known to man, and that's taking into account John Travolta's 2014 introduction of Idina Menzel at the Oscars ("Adele Dazeem" . . . who is she?). Sure, it might seem easy enough; it's just fawning, and the chances of them screwing up those first moments are slim. It's what comes *after* the initial "Aw, cute!" that strikes trepidation in visitors and puts many of them face-to-face with their fight-or-flight instincts. Yes, we're speaking of the dreaded baby hand-off.

The big problem is that (most) of you are hell-bent on having friends and family hold your babies. Or maybe you think *they* are the ones who are hell-bent. Either way, it doesn't take long after the initial "hellos" for you to extend your arms in another's direction, a baby squeezed between your hands as if you had the mobility of a Barbie doll.

Some do well with this (the ones with sensibilities for closeness, coziness, and children), which makes for a seamless transition. But for others, you might as well be handing over a spooked and clearly undomesticated chicken. It doesn't come as naturally, and their inability to accommodate the erratic movements of an infant looks even more awkward than it feels. After about thirty seconds of a two-way struggle, friends will be ready to throw the ~~chicken~~ child and run.

To be clear, no one is going to toss a baby, but moms must acknowledge the fact that some people aren't ready for that sort of physical commitment (however brief). It creates an uneasiness, and your child probably isn't having the best time, either. Often, though, the unmistakable signs of a person shying away from an armful of tot are lost on starry-eyed new moms. Even verbal refusals have a tendency of falling on deaf ears. It's as if you cannot compute a distaste for contact with your bundle of joy because who in their right mind could deny *your* child? That wasn't a rhetorical question—the answer is *anyone*, and it's nothing personal. It's merely the prerogative of the individual. So remember that though everyone is happy to *see* the baby, not everyone will be happy to invade the baby's personal space. And vice versa.

Speaking for the Baby

This happens when you decide that you *must* be a voice for your child—and not the kind that implies advocacy for those afraid to speak up on their own. Instead, it manifests as answering questions about your baby *as* your baby, as if you had one of the Sea Witch's enchanted conch necklaces hanging around your neck with his or her larynx trapped inside.

This isn't anything new; most pet owners are guilty of the exact same thing, but that doesn't make it any less warped. Think of it as introducing the alternate personality no one knew you had (and who also happens to be delightfully plagued by a speech impediment). "How is he/she?" guests may ask, to which you will answer, "Oh, he/she says, *I do-win gweat*," or "he/she says, *I'm ti-wud . . .*" This performance can make a standard visit feel like a rehearsal for the maternity ward's upcoming production of *Cybil*. Tone down the method acting, however harmless your intentions; your overzealous approach is scaring (and maybe even scarring?) everyone.

Maybe this is mom's way of bridging the communication gap between the verbal(s) and non-verbal in the room. For example, only you can tell if your dog is comfortable with a situation because you're most familiar with its mannerisms. In the same way, moms are acting interpreters for their offspring, constantly trying to open up the conversation to include all of the idiot grown-ups who don't know how to speak "newborn." Still, there will always be translations that are truly unnecessary. Phrases such as "Baby made a stinky!" or "Baby want boobies!" come to mind. Consider the advice Jillian's inner-self offered her after she convinced herself, upon leaving a spa, that her foreign bikini waxer was using the language barrier between them to make public jokes about her pubic parts: somethings are just best left misunderstood.

Easy Does It

Maybe we need to bring back those glass enclosures Depression-era researchers used to "secretly" display the Dionne Quintuplets during visiting hours. (It was later revealed by Cecile Dionne that these viewings were *not* so secret as the shadows of spectators were clearly visible to the children through a fine mesh covering, which, as you can imagine, was not disruptive or weird at all . . . .) Yes, the original idea is more than a few tweaks away from perfect, but an updated version may well prove desirable for those quaky adults. With distinct boundaries in place, the integrity of their ineptitude surrounding adult-infant interaction remains intact, and everyone involved maintains their comfort zones. And would it really be *so* bad if kids missed out on one-on-one contact with a couple of unsure strangers? The answer is always no.

At some point, everyone eventually meets the baby. Who cares if there are fumbles for the first few minutes? At least there is nowhere to go but up. Every encounter will show a modicum of improvement, and perhaps one day all the grown-ups in the baby's life will be able to throw him or her in the air while telling you (who will be rightly horrified) to "calm down" and "learn to relax." Because when the fear of the baby recedes, the fear of an angry mother will take its place. Like the way it was always meant to be.

BREASTFEEDING

They're There, They're Bare—Get Used to It!

"Breast is best" is a mantra most moms are familiar with. Know-it-all parents and nosy strangers love to rub this in the faces of those who either can't breastfeed or choose not to. Maybe you want to test the nursing waters because it helps you bond with your baby or because of its nutritional/health benefits. Or maybe your reasoning isn't clear to you at all; maybe you're going the boob route because you've cracked under societal pressures and are choosing to sacrifice your nipples to avoid being judged by the peanut gallery. Whatever your rationale, if you do decide to turn yourself into your child's own personal feeding trough, at least you can count on this chapter and those close to you for a shoulder to lean on when you need one. And you're going to need one, especially since yours are probably aching from having to hold up the two giant milk bags squished between them. Ah, the futility of the nursing bra.

Your friends may not experience the intimate issues of breastfeeding firsthand, but they will be hearing about them and will likely bear witness to them, too. The painful truth is that breastfeeding isn't always as beautiful as it's been made out to be. It's like someone has gone behind your back and signed your nipples up for the Boston Marathon when they haven't even learned to walk yet. They're going to spring leaks like a douchebag's waterbed. They're going to make surprise appearances. They may at times have strange devices strapped to them, devices that will look like they've been plucked from the set of *Mystery Science Theatre 3000*. It can be messy, uncoordinated, and awkward, kind of like losing your virginity all over again (yay . . .). And though it won't always be a calamity, it will always be, in every meaning of the word, uncomfortable. If not for you, then for somebody else. You can count on it.

Bosom Etiquette for Dummies

Let's talk straight boob talk for a minute (or a chapter). The down-and-dirty details usually left out of the Kumbaya mumbo-jumbo. Now, we like to think of ourselves and our group of friends as a pretty liberal bunch. We're free and we're chill. We're open to almost anything and hip to almost anybody. We've eaten at vegan restaurants even though we love meat, and we've even considered purchasing clothing made from organic materials (probably; you never know). There is one area, however, in which we are both admittedly not as well versed as the rest of the crew. An area we choose to very deliberately close ourselves off to. An area where we could possibly be seen as "prudish": the exposed breast area.

We've all seen our friends' boobs. Whether by accident or on purpose, every so often one or two can't help but make an appearance. That's life. But if Jillian can speak candidly for a moment, she would like readers to note that her inhibited self prefers to keep the chronicity of these events as controlled as possible. So, while everyone's whipping off their tops and bras, swapping clothes in someone's bedroom, and preparing for a Saturday night on the town, you can find her in the corner, tangled up inside a T-shirt, trying to get her arms through the armholes without exposing any side boobs or, God forbid, a nipple. Because for as long as she can remember, she has been *that friend*—the one who won't look your tits in the eyes.

That nudity makes us *both* uncomfortable is not symptomatic of any deep-rooted, stifled sexual hang-ups. We don't have mammary-envy; we're just not interested in being around your knockers and are *totally* cool with you having just as little interest in ours (of course, in Jillian's case it would be the smaller version of knockers—doorbells, perhaps?). Fortunately, we get by okay without too many people pushing their bare bods on us, trying to get us to "loosen up," but once someone gives birth, it's like being thrust between the pages of a *National Geographic* magazine—around every corner are friends' throbbing, engorged racks.

That said, nobody wants to be that person who gets grossed out by a pal feeding her baby. That's not us, and breastfeeding is *not* gross. Our complex has nothing to do with little baby what's-its-nuts. You take the child out of the equation, and we'd *still* want you to keep it in your ~~pants~~ blouse. So for the very first time ever, this can be said and meant: it really isn't you, it's us. Your breast-*feeding* isn't the issue; your breasts are. And so are her breasts and my breasts and his breasts and everyone's breasts, okay?

Give Guests Something to Look At

Even family and friends like Jillian, with all their short-comings in maturity, want to "be there" through this revealing new chapter. However, seeing you in bosom(y) buddy mode is going to take some getting used to. Much against her will, Jillian, who we mentioned regularly goes to great lengths to prevent her own indecent exposure, saw more of her sister's boobs in the first thirty-three hours after the birth of her nephew than she did in the thirty-three years she's known her, and that sister couldn't have cared less. On top of that were the times this same sibling would only halfway commit to getting dressed by throwing on a shirt and paying no mind to the buttons or clasps, swinging free and easy. It was a lot to take in, more than she had planned, but it was also more or less unavoidable because the truth is women coming off a child's birth aren't going to notice if their nudity is affecting anyone. You're too busy wearing the hell out of your newly acquired "not giving a fuck" card. But just because a person's discomfort is going unnoticed doesn't mean it's going away. So, what did Jillian do? She looked for ways to be both present and comfortable—by using the power of distraction. Anything to thwart the awkwardness that can accompany topless hangouts. And she's not the only one who has been struck by this thought . . .

Let's share a particularly amusing article we found online on WomensHealth.gov entitled "Ten things moms can do while breastfeeding." It was obvious as soon as we dove in that we had not struck oil; instead we had struck garbage. To begin with, the items were *so* not listworthy. For example, one of the top ten things to do while breastfeeding is to "Drink water." Okay, if it takes seeing it in writing for someone to know that they can indeed have a glass of water if they want a glass of water, then perhaps that person should be referring to a completely different list altogether. Something along the lines of: "Top Ten Early Signs of Dementia" or "Top Ten Reasons to Get Out More." Granted, drinking more water is supposed to help with milk supply, but you know what? So is drinking dark beer, reportedly, and between the two, that's no Sophie's Choice—you go for the dark beer.

Also making the list is the simple command "Dance," as well as "Listen to an Audiobook," which is basically just a more exciting way to say "Hear." We're surprised "Breathe" didn't crack the top five, or maybe "Be alive." And for those just dying to know what rounded out the count at number ten, here it is:

10. Cook, clean, whatever.

After scraping the bottom of the barrel and coming up with cooking and cleaning, it's as if the authors finally surrendered to the redundancy of numbers one through nine and pinched it off with the truth: "Whatever." Yes, you can do whatever, as in do nothing or do something—speak, smell, laugh, cry, or simply exist as a normal human being. After reading that, we came up with a

Top One thing the writer could do with the list. Can you guess what it is?

On top of being useless, the list also targets the wrong audience. As we've demonstrated, it's not moms who need distraction during breastfeeding sessions; they're "preoccupied" enough already. No, it's the other people in the room who need suggestions. The ones who don't know what to do with themselves. Somebody should make *them* a list so they can stop searching for new spaces on the wall to fixate their gaze upon whenever a girlfriend adjusts a left or right breast. And we did. Here are some activities that can sufficiently sidetrack your pals while you're in the middle of your one-woman burlesque show:

- Read whatever is lying around. Is that an old address book? A Chinese takeout menu? The back of a hand-sanitizing bottle? These things will never provoke more interest from guests as they do when your whole top half is hanging out of the neck hole of your shirt.
- Turn something on. Anything—a phone, a TV, a blender. Divert as many sensory organs as possible until the deafening volume of your breasts has been dialed down.

- Suggest a snack run. While indulging in your new parasitic relationship, why not nurture your symbiotic one by getting pals out of the house and into the convenience store? Who doesn't love chips and chocolate bars? By the time they get back, your baby should be fast asleep and you'll be back to your old self, fully clothed, just the way they like you.
- Let them do your dishes or tidy up, and don't feel bad about it! Friends gain brownie points, and you stay out of their sight! This is a good one.

All of this breastfeeding nonsense takes some getting used to—for everybody. Although friends can breathe a sigh of relief knowing you don't need help to manually express your milk, cringe-worthy moments will continue to crop up. Which is fine and normal. Embarrassing moments are what great friendships are built on, and trust us when we say that there's oodles of them waiting to be wrung out of breastfeeding. Enter the nursing bra!

You Bring Unsexy Back (Yeah!)

Everyone knows what one of these looks like, right? If not, picture your mom's bras. You know, the ones that were very obviously purchased in the seventies and seem to have been sold exclusively in only two shades:

"Cigarette Yellow" and "Decades of Sweat." It is this imagery that many minds wander to whenever a nursing bra comes up in conversation—a worn-and-weary bra that needs to be sent back (in time) to the Macy's warehouse where it came from.

Thankfully, modern versions have undergone some much-needed improvements and are a far cry from the atrocities they had strapped onto baby boomers. Even the bare bones of the design are more suited for the female form, instead of the set of cow udders older models seemed to have been marketed toward. Basically, you have these ordinary, kind-of-ugly bras that, at some point during creation, were hijacked by snaps, hooks, and secret passageways. What the hell is this? A negligée or a really uncool Swiss army knife for the previously unarmed chest?

Maybe this is one of those times when looks don't matter. These things aren't built for speed or aesthetics; they're built for utility—it says right in the name "nursing bra." But utilitarian or not, it's still a bra that comes not just off but also *apart*, allowing the operator to play peek-a-boo with boobs: flaps come up and down, breasts pop in and out. You'd think these bad boys would be driving men (or women) wild, and at the rate new moms are feeding their babies, how *aren't* partners in a constant state of hot and heaviness? But the unfortunate truth of the matter is that bras with built-in holes do not ooze the same amounts of sex appeal as their counterpart, the crotch-less panty. Despite the underwear with the bottoms cut out are big sellers in the XXX stores, nursing bras just cannot seem to spark the same fire; instead, they are fire repellant, like big stretchy nylon fire extinguishers.

It could always be worse, and you probably don't want to breastfeed dressed as some scantily-clad coquettish ingénue anyway. It's "Sexy Nurse," not "Sexy *Wet Nurse*," and let's face it, those boobs don't need a cup-less, snap-crotch teddy to look like they belong in the red-light district. It how they're plated—their size will overshadow, or eclipse, anything working against them. Never, ever underestimate the power of the rack.

The Cost of Big Boobs

Big is great. Big is the bee's knees. But there's always going to be downsides to your double-edged set of naturally occurring, temporary implants. Remember that milk isn't going to stick around forever; at some point, the wells will run dry. Not to mention the fact that breastfeeding can also, in a word, suck—sometimes *so* hard that you won't be able to do it exclusively, or at all. Maybe you think, *Big deal*, or *Super, now I can drink*; but the road toward those laissez-faire attitudes is not without frustrations; too much milk; not enough milk; milk slow to come in; milk that never comes. Bad latch. Sore nipples; cracked nipples; chapped nipples; nipples caked in blood. And we'll stop there because it's beginning to sound like we're moving away from potentially problematic side-effects and into ingredients fit for a witch's cauldron.

At some point, the physical demand mixed with the lack of sleep and seesawing emotions are going to wear on you. They will manifest into tears, and your partner's ear may not necessarily be your first choice to bend all your feelings over. Maybe you need to cry about your boobs to someone with an empathetic pair, a breast friend to play Detective Google with to nullify any deep-rooted fears that your nipples have a real chance of falling off from all the unrelenting tugging. Or maybe you just need them to pass you the chafing cream with a knowing look that says "Yes, your baby is being an asshole right now, but maybe someday he or she will be famous." Because along with communicating with single glances, squad members also specialize in the verbalization of what you need to hear until things improve, or at least until the baby scrams. It always has been and will be their job to help you soldiering on, no matter how sticky the wicket.

Milk and Formula

Can you guess which members of your inner circle drank breast milk as a baby versus those who drank formula? No, you can't. That's because of all the variables that affect whether or not people develop into functional members of society, none are dependent on the ability to form a good latch. But these days, moms who choose to feed their babies formula face a lot of criticism. If you're one of these women, you've got to be ready to fight. Just as with breastfeeding, there are reasons women choose to feed with formula—Baby will sleep more and eat less, and Mom will have more freedom. And to further your cause, a bunch of smart people in lab coats have made it their mission to certify that formula is nutritious! In fact, if they were to make an updated version of *The Grapes of Wrath*, we are sure the woman at the end of the book could have just as effectively nursed that half-starved man with a bottle as she did her boob. Different impact for the reader, same outcome for the desperate man in need. Powerful stuff!

Alternatively, going the traditional route means you're going to have a baby on your boob all day and all night. You need to practice mindful defense against the agoraphobia that will try and take hold. Never leaving the house so you can easily whip one out for Baby can turn even the most outgoing women into shut-ins. So even if your new nudist tendancies give friends the heebie-jeebies, and the animalistic snorting and grunting noises that accompany suckling bring about unwanted attention, breastfeeding in public is normal and necessary. So, don't be shy—chances are many of your friends are ready and waiting to hand out beatdowns to any jerk-off who hints that a nursing woman's place is in her home. Putting terrible people back in their place is an axe that feels so good to grind. If the Spice Girls albums taught us anything, it's never give up an opportunity to kick-ass in the name of girl power.

Your New Normal

Congratulations on your new career as "Lactation Distribution Jockey Extraordinaire." Not everyone gets the chance to make meals with parts of their body. That's a privilege reserved for only the finest Mother Nature has to offer—moms (and those girls from "2 Girls 1 Cup"). You've come quite a long way, from being someone we assume was *never* above pissing behind nightclubs to someone who is a caretaker and provider of the highest caliber. And with these new powers, know that if anyone ever runs out of cream for their coffee, there is a human dairy dispenser at their fingertips!

Breast- or bottle-feeding, milk or formula, proceed however you see fit. Switch it up or stick with one, and let people who cannot help themselves draw their own unfair conclusions if they must. Because you are above that now. You're a mom.

THE BIRTH STORY
The Best That TMI Has to Offer

It's pretty common for outsiders to ask for the birth story, but what's even more common is getting the birth story without asking. Oversharing is something that gets turned *way* up postpartum—just ask any mom's Facebook account. Somewhere between the first contraction and last stitch, mothers figured any individual who wasn't front, row, and center during delivery must be dying for the gruesome play-by-play, whether it be through a series of obscene oral recollections or crude imagery plastered across social media.

For all the places and times these stories can be relived appropriately, there are a million more where they cannot. Know these boundaries, like the way Allison knows we can only bring up "The Purse Story" (an unfortunate dilemma involving Jillian, an intestinal need, and a toilet refusing to flush) when there are no male ears present. Or the way no woman, during her annual performance review, would ever mention that time she went to remove her tampon and found two strings instead of the usual one. This is because stories centered around objects being removed from the human body (i.e., warts, kidneys, feminine products, or babies) are rated R for a reason. But moms have, many times over, chosen to cast these restrictions aside, adopting and implementing their own unapproved rating system, which has only one tier: E for Everyone.

However you spin your stories, you can't always separate something unpleasant from its unpleasantness. Think of how expiration date works on all that chocolate almond milk you continue to buy but can never seem to finish. Even if you fudge the "best before" numbers in the name of "waste-not-and-want-not"ing (or to save yourself from another trip to 7-11), you're not going to dislike any less what's festering inside the carton.

The truth is only a handful of people are interested in the nitty-gritty of childbirth, and out of that group, maybe half can stomach it. We're not saying you should bury all memories of your delivery deep within yourself, only to reveal them years later while splayed across a chaise lounge in your therapist's office; we're just saying that the deck of cards you have now isn't one everyone wants to play with. Be conscious in your dealing. That means no spinning yarns to your hairstylist, your little brother's girlfriend, your grandmother's church group, or the person in front of you at the supermarket checkout. They haven't had nearly enough prep to handle such hazardous material.

But if you're desperate for a pair of ears to take away on your vagina's expedition from sex organ to mincemeat, you have your BFFs. That's what they're for, *especially* if they are the child-free sort. Think about it, they don't have a tale like this to call their own. If they're curious for the gory details, they're left relying on said mommy pals. It is because of close friends like Allison that Jillian knows how truly macabre labor can be (let's just say her vomit-filled adventure did *not* involve a blow-out like you've seen on *Friends* or overwritten, playful jibber-jabber as shown on *Gilmore Girls*). As one friend recalls, it can involve scrambling on all fours in front of strangers, while you scream internally, *I'm going to shit myself. I'm going to shit myself. Will they tell me if I'm shitting myself?* As another so matter-of-factly puts it: "My *ass* fell out . . . of itself. Who *does* that?" They're right; it's madness. It makes *The Human Centipede* look like an innocent game of leapfrog. But it's real life, and if your *tightest* friends are anything like us, they are going to want to hear this story almost as badly as you're dying to tell it.

A Version for Friends/A Version for Everyone Else

Looking at the way birth stories are brandished, we're surprised mothers haven't jumped to the scripted door-to-door solicitation routine, a la the Jehovah's Witnesses: "Do you have a moment? Today, I would like to share with you the good word that is my birth story." Don't put it past them—a mom's target demographic, if you ask her, is the entire planet. Still, childbirth is a high stakes game and one vagina-load of an undertaking. Some describe it as a "one-in-a-million" experience, others lean toward "near death." Whatever side you're on, the after buzz is sure to drive you to overshare, like the way people practically orgasm when reminiscing about an epic fight: the adrenaline starts pumping, and before you know it you're shadowboxing by yourself in your living room while everyone else at the party has moved to the kitchen. This is what can happen if you allow yourself to get caught up in your own story, while all the people you thought were listening will slowly pull away.

At the risk of sounding like a couple of cantankerous harridans, you need to ix-nay the indecent proposals or at least vet your audience before you unleash them. You'll know they are qualified if they have at one time (or many times) witnessed you in a "period through the jeans" situation, *or* if they have a casual familiarity with your current stance on anal sex. In fact, that last one should be considered the benchmark when it comes to birth stories: unless both participants can recount the other's sexual butt history *from memory*, they aren't ready to discuss all the bloody by-products of procreation.

This means you should equip yourself with two versions of the same tale. Version A (for Appalling) will be the unabridged version, i.e., the one for the women described above. It should include all the fecal matters, how much of the perineum was salvaged, how you go about wiping yourself now that you've basically had a meteor blow through you, etc. This version is the kind that gal pals might want to pop some popcorn for and also slap on one of your life-raft-sized postpartum maxi pads, because the ensuing laughter will cause the peeing of many pants.

Version B (for Benign) is for "other people," the "adorable" version, candy-coated to give those on the receiving end cavities. You're going to need to edit out anything that happened between your first superhuman push and when you are handed your baby. Leave all the blood, sweat, and amniotic fluid on the cutting room floor. Then, test what's left on your most uptight grandmother, the one who still makes all the unmarried adult couples sleep in separate rooms and draws offense from the use of *darn* in a sentence. If she can get from beginning to end feeling all warm and fuzzy, as opposed to nauseated and retching, you've found your actual "E for Everyone."

The One Thing Women Really Want to Know

It's always a joy finding articles on the Internet that are obviously the result of a freelance copywriter trying to hit a deadline. It's those situations that lead to articles like this one, published on the website *nursingbirth.com* in 2009: "Top 10 Dos & DON'Ts of Pooping During Labor & Birth."

We have so many questions, the most burning one being how did the author miss the opportunity to turn this compilation of *dos and don'ts* into *doo doos and don'ts*? That oversight is grounds for termination. Besides, are they really telling us that there are "do's" when it comes to pooping during labor? And let's not ignore the fact that "do" is pluralized! Yes, we all have our own histories of bypassing a bathroom when nature calls at a bad time, but no matter where you are and no matter what you're doing, public defecation always has been and will be a unanimous *don't*. They might as well have written a "dos and don'ts" list for ripping a huge fart in an elevator, or having a boob fall out during a PTA meeting. There is just no upside to some situations, and the only "do" that could work here would be "Do avoid whenever possible"—which is just a wordier version of "don't."

Nobody wants to shit, period, but it's not only a risk during labor; it's also almost a guarantee. Even though that might not bring a smile to your face, it will to the faces of those around you. You see, there's something about the visual of you in this savage predicament that will fill friends (like Jillian) with a childlike glee. Perhaps it's because deep within the bowels of our souls, we find the mortification and humiliation of others, especially those closest to us, hysterical. Whatever the reason, friends want to know how the poop happened, when it happened, what was felt during and after, and who saw, cared, or cares now.

Stop getting so embarrassed. This can't be the first time feces has made its way into your repartee, and it likely won't be the last. If you are one of those who tends to shy away from toilet talk, stop! You are doing your BFFs a damn disservice! This is hilarity in its purest form. Don't be ashamed if you've cleared that hurdle. Public excretion is not for the faint of heart, and even though you may still be feeling a little traumatized by it all, remember that while laughter may not be the best medicine, at least it's free.

What, This Old Thing?

The placenta—or, as we like to call it, "the conversation pariah"—is everywhere right now, polluting blog posts, Facebook walls, and Instagram feeds with its flaccid, bloody form. Moms are not only using their words to describe their after-birth; they are also now uploading pictorial representations to social media accounts, making a regular perusal of one's newsfeed feel like you've been unwillingly locked inside your butcher's deep freeze.

We're not afraid of the placenta, and we don't mind hearing about one here and there in appropriate circumstances (which almost exclusively occur while one is away from the computer). Any woman can shoot the breeze on flattened, circular transitory organs but that doesn't mean we're all rooting for an earful or, God forbid, an eyeful. A verbal acknowledgment of this uterine castaway no longer pushes the envelope hard enough for some moms, which is how unsuspecting friends end up having to "Like" these bulbous post-op masses when all they want to do is share their latest selfie.

What's with the brazen "TMI"? Are women worried we're not "buying" their birth stories as truth, and as a result tack on raunchy visuals to prove they did, in fact, deliver? We're not talking about Beyoncé here; it's not like there have been whispers of surrogacy. So put down the camera and your placenta, for Christ's sake! We believe you! We believe you!

You Are Woman. We Are, Too.

But maybe it's to prove something else. Listen, if any of these inclinations have anything to do with the "I am woman, hear me roar" mentality, then you have it all wrong. If Allison had posted her placenta on Facebook, she would do about as much for the feminist movement as Jillian would by posting a picture of her used maxi-pad as a way to demonstrate her barren condition. We refuse to believe it makes us any less of an advocate for females if a few (or rather, the majority) of us find the wake of labor on a public forum off-putting. We're just the type of people who see a clear difference between breaking boundaries and being bush league. And if anyone feels our opinion is anti-feminist or the residual expressions of unseen patriarchal oppression, believe us when we say: it has nothing to do with that and more to do with the fact that pushing organic waste onto your social network is like Gretchen Wieners trying to push *fetch* on Regina George. Stop trying to make fetch happen. It's not going to happen.

Try Not to, But You Might

Maybe you were already aware of these drawn lines, in which case you won't have to police the thoughts and feelings making their way through your internal filter and into the outside world. Armed with either your previous or newfound self-awareness, you can now confidently unload all the graphic language and landscapes of childbirth on the right people, the ones who are comfortable with the content and, most important, the source, taking an otherwise totes inappropes birth story and turning it into a big figurative bowl of Lucky Charms: magically delicious. And if you catch yourself getting carried away, maybe while captioning a photo of your baby's head beginning to crown, step away from your computer, drop the smartphone, and give yourself the talk. The talk that we just had. Verbatim, if that helps.

THE MATERNAL
URGE TO BLOG

*You Are Going to Become a Writer,
and You Better Be the Worst*

O nce the third trimester has come and gone, you will slowly but surely begin shifting gears. Over the past few months, you've focused your total attention on being prepared and able (albeit apprehensively) to spring into parenting at any moment. Driven by pre-traumatic stress and your typical strain of everyday anxiety, there was one task at hand: to get the proverbial pre-baby ducks into a perfect little row before the big day. And look at that, you've pulled it off. Almost.

You've purchased a car seat at a cost that could have covered your first year of university and played master designer during the creation of the most Pinterest-worthy nursery ever. You've bombed around from store to store, stocking up on the little things: diapers for baby, "diapers" for mommy (aka extra thick overnight pads), nipple guards, nipple creams, and a donut-shaped horror whose sole purpose is to alleviate the discomfort that comes along with a baby blowing through a woman as if her swimsuit area were made of perforated parchment paper.

Now you're exactly where you need to be, and the dust that blew up after your crash-landing into motherhood is settling. It sure would be nice to sit back and let the bonding play out like a sickeningly sweet Regina Spektor album—but you're a mom now. You're never "sitting back" again, and since you're up, there is something you could get a jump on. A must-have for every newbie in today's Internet-fueled parenting world and the only sure-fire way to secure your contention for World's ~~Most Vainglorious~~ Greatest Mom—your very own, totally unwarranted Mommy Blog.

What the $%@! is a Mommy Blog Anyway?

For some moms, a blog is platform for your own catharsis by sharing day-to-day peaks and troughs, however broad or personalized. For the less vocal, they are sources of relatable material where one can find relief or, for more frivolous searches, their daily dose of the ever persistent and highly exhausted "mom and wine joke."

Jillian has been looking for an in on this scene for some time, but since Allison would rather die than become another self-appointed prophet for parents, she's had to settle for the thoughts and feelings of strangers as opposed to the public preaching of someone close to her (and, for the record, so has Allison—just because you're not writing your own doesn't mean you're not reading everyone else's). The Mommy Blog, specifically the sort written by women who enlist themselves the moment their parenting cherry is popped, is basically a glorified online journal that details the ins and outs of child-rearing *as interpreted by the writer*. Remember that last bit when you embark on your quest to find your blogess-counterpart and are not immediately dazzled by what you discover. These blogs may be everywhere, but they can't all be condensed versions of Oprah's *Lifeclass*.

Pervasiveness does have its upsides, though. The number of options available to you, and the variety within them, really does widen the goalposts. As mentioned, many of these blogs bring tremendous value for readers who are looking for substantial connections and take-aways. They have been executed with thoughtfulness, humor, and an honest approach to maternal triumphs and perceived failures. It's too bad, then, that this is a chapter where we wade into the shallowest of depths.

We're not interested in blogs that offer admirable, qualitative analyses on parenting; we're only concerned with the blogs that have been executed . . . period. The weirdest and the worst of Mommy Blogging. Not because we're trying to drag down the cause, but because some of these things need to be said and some of these jokes have to be made. The upregulation of Mommy Blogs wills it so. We'll also show you how to use these notes to get your own half-assed contribution up and running because, as you probably know, Mommy Bloggers are a lot like family doctors—if you can't find one you like, just become your own . And before you ask yourself "Should I?," flip the question to "Can I?" If you apply our advice provided below purely for the sake of your amusement, the answer will be a resounding *yes*.

All Aboard?

Nobody forgets you've been through hell and back to birth your baby, and taking on a project—especially one that you were unqualified for just weeks before—may not have been part of your plan going forward. Besides, what kind of unabashed person takes advantage of their new mom status, anyway? Who dare use it as a license to write, share, and promote their self-conceited parenting wins as if the only requirements for PhD grade expertise were to "Parent Hard Daily"? The answer is everyone. Everyone does/did/is/has/will. It's not like you weren't already exploiting the hell out of your pregnancy—parking in the maternity space next to the grocery store entrance while the urine was still drying on your EPT, shamelessly wringing crocodile tears out onto your super-sized belly to get out of that speeding ticket, and canceling the dinner your friends planned six weeks in advance because the kettle chips told you to. Is blogging "just because you can" *that* big a leap from your usual tricks? No, and we are *so* here for it!

But maybe you're not worried about abusing your power—or the mediocre content. Maybe it's the time issue that's conflicting you. How can you stand behind wild declarations of busyness if you're stealing moments to build and stoke a fire under an online following? Won't shamers allege that hours devoted to blogging could be better spent connecting with your child? Maybe, but everyone will always have a bone to pick in one capacity or another, no matter how much attention you pay to your kids. So here's what you should tell them (with a self-determined amount of sarcasm): Mommy Blogs are not, as some cynics might say, just gratuitous expressions of self-importance and praise. They can be much, much more.

(Why and) How to Get Started

To be considered the real deal, you must meet only one key prerequisite: you must be a mother. That's it. You don't need to be a good mother or a good writer, for that matter. You don't need experience (in the literary or parenting sense), and you certainly don't need to know what you're talking about. All that's required is a pulse, a birthing event, and an Internet connection. And in terms of commitment, don't worry—everyone dedicates the time they have based on the schedule they keep, which we've broken down into two distinct categories:

Group A: Moms who update on a regular basis. These are women who have something child-free folk like to refer to as "spare moments." They have the money to hire a nanny while still being able to dish out for dozens of diapers per week, and the extra set of hands grants them access to the ever elusive "window of personal time" on the daily. These are the moms who always *say* they're busy, but the reality is they're drowning in help. In short, these are the fully-grown, spoiled brat moms (demographic with which our generation is exceptionally lousy).

Group B: On the flip side, we have the "regular mom" types. They are much more preoccupied than their devil-may-care, cash-happy counterparts, and they have a better chance of finding a passage to Narnia in the bottom of their diaper bags than stumbling across a minute alone. If this mom plans on becoming a "writer girl" (a term coined by America's national *treasure* train wreck Aviva Drescher and past "Real Housewife of New York City"), she will have to rely on the gaps in someone else's calendar to get things off the ground (pregnant women aren't supposed to lift anyway, right?). This is where friends can serve their purposes, probably eagerly and absolutely hilariously.

It's called ghostwriting. It won't matter that it isn't you physically typing or that it's not necessarily your personal outlook or voice. The most important thing is that *someone* is sending something—~~anything~~—out into the webiverse often enough to create a buzz, all the while keeping in mind the golden rule of Mommy Blogging: when it comes to sharing moments nobody has asked for, do it as publicly and frequently as humanly possible. Once your pinch prosateur has you a couple posts deep and the benefits start to outweigh the costs, you can move forward, unaided. And don't worry about alpha readers to proof your latest travesty. Friends aren't responsible for cleaning up your literary mess. You shouldn't want them to, anyway. Why screw with imperfection? They can, however, prove useful once the comments start rolling in and you need a partner to relish in the mislead love or hard-earned haters.

Finding a Catchy Name

This is where you'll really see the creative juices ooze, like puss from a gangrenous limb begging to be amputated—but don't cut it off just yet. When it comes to the blogosphere, your ideas may be worth saving. Think of all the moms you know, the archetypes. Now imagine those archetypal blog names. Whatever comes to mind likely already exists, and a light Google search will reveal similar "high-grade" intellectual property that has, against all odds, been claimed. Everything from *Mommy Poppins*, which is not without the implications of "having and doing it all" (a type of woman Candice Bergen declared to "hate" during a Barbara Walters interview) to *The Trophy Wifestyle*, is "having it all while doing nothing." Then there's our personal favorite, *The Mommy Files*, which should be a fan-fiction site surrounding a hypothetical scenario where Agent Dana Scully keeps her alien baby and raises it inside the walls of the United States Federal Bureau of Investigation. But it's not; it's just another mommy blog (and honestly, even under its new name *Redhead Mom*, it's not too shabby).

Within these examples are distinct underpinning flavors of brashness and unapologetic spunk. If you plan to attract the online sassy mom traffic, you'll need just the right words with just the right amount of mojo representing you and your virtual domain. One way to begin this process is by "Vision Board-ing," which involves sparking inspiration by ruining your favorite magazines in order to make a collage barely fit for a third grade art fair. But if you'd like to avoid massacring your gossip rags or hanging the visual testimony of your creative limits above your desk, you can always go back to basics with a classic brainstorming session.

Now, we're not sure how they did things in America in the early nineties, but in the Canadian public school system, all you needed to stir up a brainstorm was a pencil and a piece of paper. First, you illustrate a little cloud with the core subject written inside.

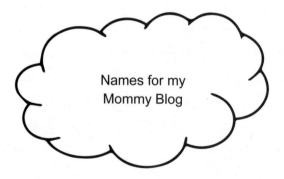

Then, you draw lines about the perimeter. The more ambitious you are, the more lines you will need:

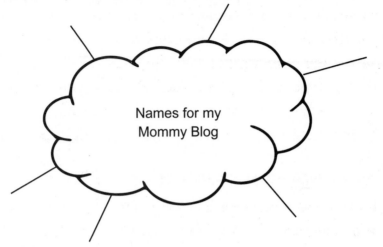

Lastly and most important, you attach potential solutions to the end of each line.

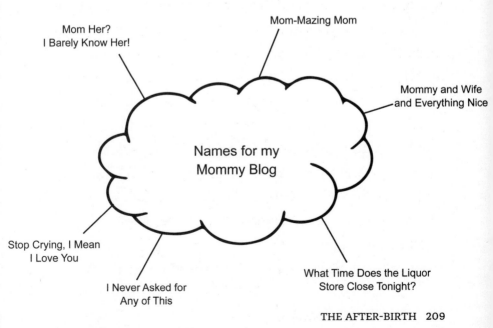

As you can see, it can be hard to stay focused. Give it a shot, and by the time you're finished, you should have something that resembles the stick-cloud hybrid above or, when sketched free-hand, a poorly drawn porcupine surrounding by chicken scratch. Once you are face-to-face with your juicy "mind grapes" (thank you, *30 Rock*), it's as easy as choosing whatever stands out the most and running with it as quickly and carelessly as possible.

Antagonization through Imagery

Don't assume a blog's success relies solely on content or a killer name. Just as significant, if not more so, is the corresponding imagery, which most often features the stars of the show: you and baby. Finding the right pictorial tone for a Mommy Blog involves more than just a snap-and-go approach. Done properly, these images will provide viewers who lap up kitten videos on YouTube with their daily dose of figurative cheese. Done improperly, though, they can end up looking like rejected stock photos, and the last thing you want is *your* blog looking like a second-rate Kmart catalog. It's virtual suicide.

Similar missteps can be avoided with a little foresight and a lot of A-Game. For instance, since becoming a blogger usually means becoming a model, you need some dependably slay-able poses to ease you into the spotlight. A classic over-the-shoulder head shot is a safe way for a novice like yourself to make, well, not "your" mark, but "a" mark nevertheless. It takes a minimal amount of effort to turn one's head slightly to the left or right, and it's better to start out beige than slip off into the deep end too soon and drowning in your own contrived glamour.

The Art of Being Bad

Even if you are killing it on all levels, you may be underwhelmed by the amount of hits and/or feedback churned out each week. It's not your fault. The blogs drawing in the big crowds are home-runs in either genius or disaster (and remember, we're aiming you for door number two). Our favorite blogs to scroll through are ones that make our brains feel under siege—the ones in dire need of linguistic defibrillation, the ones marred with the sort of verbal carnage that leaves one's inner masochist thirsty for more. If reading the first few paragraphs creates an insatiable urge to reach through the computer and slap the writer, then she has done her job. Basically, it's time to dumb yourself down, if only for the sake of notoriety, and if you didn't pick up on that a few sentences back, you might not have much work ahead of you!

Being good at being bad has never been this fun. Most of us, young and old, have managed to suck at many things in our lifetimes—relationships, cooking, frisbee golf, real golf, plant ownership, parallel parking, and, of course, blogging. Whether it be a series of estranging paragraphs or a well-placed run-on sentence, a firm underestimation of the public's intelligence, shown in the examples below, cannot miss.

- An utter disregard for the English language will stop any reader dead in his or her tracks. This method is a personal favorite, and it can be a blast. To most people, confusing *there, their,* and *they're,* in a world with spell-check, is unforgivable, especially when you're meant to be, you know, somewhat of a writer (well, *blogger*). But typos and grammatical screwups are the foundation of your magnum opus. So, kick everything you learned in language arts to the curb and toss your dictionary in the trash. You won't be needing them anymore.

- Consistently adding nothing new to the blog world is irritating. That is, recycling unoriginal topics with an even less original touch. There is nothing intriguing about reading cliché rhetoric where the reader can anticipate the author's next move word for word. For example, this sentence: "My daughter's first day of school; where does the time go? Heart is melting." Why not personalize this event by sharing an embarrassing moment or humanizing your family dynamic, i.e., "My daughter's first day of school, and I can't get off the john. #colitis!" That's a nail-biter.

- Unsourced or poorly sourced medical advice is a great way to get the brighter half of an audience seething (and the dimmer half nodding in agreement at every word). That is, taking on some "think piece" by a non-doctor at another parenting blog as fact, as opposed to say, you know, referencing facts. "This disorder can be regulated by increasing fruit and vegetable intake and is frequently misdiagnosed." These are just words; anyone can type them (we just did). People hate being told how to heal their children by someone who is just as unqualified as they are. If they were after the uneducated opinion of an ordinary person, they would be showing up at friends' doorsteps when their kids catch a cold instead of the local clinic. So, anytime you want to put your match into that tinderbox they call a comment section, drop some off-the-cuff health tips based on nothing.

Remember, to really piss people off, you must never acknowledge any of your blunders and never, ever edit for the sake of improvement after a post goes live. The goal is to provoke to the point of offline discussion, where readers will tell their friends and their friends will tell their friends, and soon everyone is swinging by your web address trying to break your code-like illiteracy.

Tack on a Theme (The Five F's)

Not that you have much of a choice, but mothers tend to pull their subject matter from their life experiences alone, confusing it to be of universal interest to others. The reality is a shit taken by your baby, though it may be the highlight of your afternoon, won't often evoke the same excitement in others. Not that writing about the sedulous efforts of growing and birthing babies isn't great, but it has a limited reach. There is no momentum when the topic of conversation is confined to the same infant. That's why the most successful blogs squeeze more out of their online airtime than just parenting advice and corresponding anecdotes. And how do they reach the masses? By adding a theme, that's how.

This extra angle is key. It's what you make time for when you're *not* caring for baby that determines your sub-niche. And if you're unsure of what you want to claim as your "passion," here are a few popular motifs commonly associated with Mommy Blogs:

Fitness Mommy: No one is as jazzed to re-start their workout regimens as "Fitness Mommy." You're tired. You want a nap. And a lobotomy. You don't want to bounce your heaving shoulder-boulders around, trying to keep track of your new post-birth body parts while following along with a thirty-minute workout DVD. However, if you are exercise-savvy and you have the will and the way to get in shape post-baby, then this is a sure-fire way to get on everyone's last nerve.

Faith-Happy Mommy: Faith is sewn, however delicately or heavily, into the fabric of every Mommy Blog. Most of it is blind, but some is religious and can be perplexing for non-bible thumpers. That being said, if your worship and parenting are that intertwined, you are probably expecting a like-minded audience. Not that it matters, but it probably wouldn't include us. Unless you're into Scientology. Those documentaries aren't messing around, and we desperately want to know how and when exactly President Xenu came between Joey Potter and Tom Cruise.

Fashion Mommy: Out of all the types of blogs, we hate this one the most. Outfit of the day? Is there any other kind? And why does every one of these women own a wool cape? And who buys a toddler Hunter rain boots?

They're, like, one hundred dollars! Do you know how it makes adults feel when the three-year-old at Starbucks is in rain gear worth more than your entire ensemble? Damn you, Fashion Mommy, and your best dressed mini-me.

Food Mommy: This is the mom everyone wants to have around, one who still hasn't shaken her serious case of the munchies. Food is what unites us. We all want it, we need it, we love it—pizza, Taco Bell, etc. Women who have recently given birth are experienced eaters. Many spent the better part of a year chowing down, so you would think their food blogs would just be lists upon lists of ways to cheat on your diet and what bag of chips complements which flavor of shame. But it's not as cut-and-dried as you may think. Some moms are stuck-the-*F*-up. They may leave the delivery room with their bodies less one baby, but a solid rod seems to have made its way up their asses. If you want to use food to frustrate, preach organic shopping, dietary restrictions, costly substitutions, and healthy habits with zero room for alternatives. You want to emulate the tone-deafness of Gwyneth Paltrow when she said, "I would rather *die* than let my kid eat Cup-a-Soup." That was in 2005, and we're still talking about it, which goes to show how long people hold on to the ostracizing words of rotten individuals who happen to become moms.

All Crap Things Must Come to an End

Think of this chapter as a verbose guide on how to color outside of the lines while you play Mommy of the Year across computers everywhere. Even though it won't take your mind completely off motherhood, it can pull you out of the day-to-day routine that some new moms have difficulty getting used to. However good, bad, or illegible, your Mommy Blog is something just for you. *You* can create your own deadlines, *you* can storyboard, and *you* can get lost in any topic you want (as opposed to usual stresses like baby's sleeping and feeding schedules). And when you're writing in the hopes of being contemptible, you get to dick around as much or as little as you see fit. And don't worry about polishing up a technique; you don't need one. Writing your blog is about assuming the position of expert *without* possessing the expertise; it is not a place to waste extra efforts. Phone it in, and when no one answers, let the motherfucker ring.

THE MOMMY GROUP

Abandon Hope, All Ye Who Enter Here

Perhaps you feel like the friendship between you and your girlfriends has become a little, or even severely, disjointed during the past nine (plus) months. Maybe it's becoming harder and harder to get them on board with all the new "hobbies" you've picked up during your transition from being a person just like them to being a person with *actual* responsibilities. Or maybe you're becoming a bit of a snooze, and your verbal exchanges are struggling to keep their signature spark. It makes sense. It can't be easy letting go of the unfiltered shallowness that can only be found in daily discussions with close friends, but people are now telling you that those inane chats are "not what's important anymore." Instead, moms like you *must* focus on acquainting themselves with the new baby as well as the new "you"—one who is made up predominantly of emotions and bodily fluids, both of which can be seen steadily pouring from your bloodshot eyeballs (and your tits).

Sounds rough, but don't throw in the conversational towel just yet. You are sitting on a gossip gold mine, and you don't even know it. Yes, you hold the key to the potential shit show of potential shit shows—all you need to do is sign away your soul (and a few hours every few weeks), sit back, and wait for it to unravel before your eyes (and, later, friends' ears). We're talking, of course, about the Mommy group. The Mommy Shaming Olympics. The place where the passive-aggressive parenting police go to passive-aggressively police parents. So, move over, Patient Six of *General Hospital*, or whoever you are this week with all your musculature and never-changing hairstyle—it's time to make room for the *real* soap opera stars . . .

What Are Mommy Groups?

Sometimes called "playgroups" or "meet-ups," the Mommy Group is a powerful, cult-like force to be reckoned with. Yes, the moniker sounds better suited for a washed-up, over-forties acapella group destined to be sent packing during the first-round auditions of *American Idol* (is that show still relevant?), but their true purpose is to provide groups of moms with, you know, "support."

Let's examine support groups for a moment. Typically, they are non-toxic and therapeutic environments where people can find solace in relatability to others, regardless of how strange the circumstances, i.e., United Bronies of Tuscon (real), and the Alien Abductions Support Group in London (real). Mommy groups aren't *that* different—they introduce the joy of children (children with lungs capable of creating volumes that will challenge any normal decibel reach for the human voice). Members are granted access to an open forum of discussion as well as an opportunity to relieve their child-rearing struggles by amplifying their successes through the pandering of other parents.

Luckily, it doesn't have to be as terrible as it sounds. If anything, it sounds like it could be the steady boost of encouragement a lot of moms like you need and deserve, especially during those first few months when it's not uncommon to feel vulnerable or experience waves of self-doubt. And as an added advantage, this can be a perfect platform to begin your re-introduction to the social scene. But proceed with caution and remember the wise words of whoever it was who first said the words "It sounds too good to be true." It all comes down to how willing you are to take some bitter with your sweet. Maybe a lot of bitter.

Circle of Frenemies

Let's do the math: X amount of women, with X amount of points of view (yes, if this sounds familiar it *is* the old intro to Barbara Walters' five-piece hen-house program). From this equation, we can deduce that the Mommy Group experience will likely unfold for you in one of two ways:

1. You could end up tapping into a source of emotional and psychological support from other mothers in a safe and controlled setting.
2. . . . or you could end up reliving the high school experience.

Now there are many women, regardless of their place in the pecking order of grade school, who would say that these two examples are mutually exclusive. Not quite so, in the off-paper Mommy Group experience, which has the beshitted reputation for being two-faced. This is where shades of petty high school dynamics begin to creep back into your life (unless you're still in high school, in which case you should be reading other books. Real books. Helpful books).

Do not allow this possibility to deter you from joining one. Although we acknowledge that there are those among us who would gladly opt for a vaginal biopsy at a learning hospital over revisiting their freshman, sophomore, or senior years, one should not automatically dismiss an opportunity for a do-over. Remember, high school brought more to the table than just bitchy, fresh-off-puberty A-holes; it also brought with it the careless discourse of immature youth and superfluous head games. Who doesn't miss that?

It happens every time. Whenever you throw a bunch of personalities together in one room, sooner or later they are going to wear on each other regardless of age or however cavalier their reason for being there. Take for instance those heydays back when you were enrolled in Girl Scouts. On the surface, there were young ladies in uniform, wearing sashes, collecting badges based on good Samaritan-ism, and singing around campfires. But underneath that convincing mask of civic duty lay a tween-age melodrama. Tears. Cliques. Talking behind backs. Stabbing in those same backs. This will always be the Girl Scouts Jillian remembers. (Allison wouldn't understand; she dodged the scout draft when she was instead made to attend lessons in the unsung hero of all instruments, the recorder, proving once and for all that sometimes even winners can be losers.) Does Jillian recall any of the badges she earned? No. Does she remember specifically who called her "Big Nose" on a trip to Newfoundland in 1996? Yes, yes, she does. Now, tack on twenty years, and Mommy Group members still experience never-ending sinusoidal-wave-like mood fluctuations. Watch the politeness fade faster than that initial good impression you made on your significant other's parents before you poured your third double vodka, but sign up anyway—the entertainment value alone will outweigh the catty subtext . . . most of the time.

Types of Mommy Groups

Much like the Hells Angels (or *exactly* like the Hells Angels), the mommy sort are subcategorized based on specific variables. First, they are broken down according to location, and then further separated into pointlessly distinct niches. These can be of a broad variety, for example, Working Moms of Chicago and Romanian Moms of Houston (both valid chapters). They can also be incredibly obscure. For instance, in a busy metropolitan area like Manhattan, it wouldn't be totally nuts for an expectant mother to have no trouble recruiting women for factions as peculiar as, say, Single Moms Who Papier-Mâché (with Duplicates) or Stay-at-Home Moms with Three-Fingered Step-Children. So if you're in a very specific parental position, don't worry about having to reach out *too* far to find others just like you. If a group doesn't exist yet, you can always start your own. May we suggest something along the lines of Moms Looking to Dysfunction to Pacify Boredom or Women with Children Who Hate Other Women with Children.

Another way moms like to create fragmentation among themselves is by having open Mommy Groups (the welcoming sort) versus closed Mommy Groups (the unwelcoming sort). You would have no chance at a closed group. If someone were to take Mommy Groups and break them down into a "cafeteria seating chart"-esque way, these groups would be the Plastics (we know, another *Mean Girls* reference). These bitches don't believe any new member can improve on what they have already put together, so, their loss. No need to waste your time barking up conceited trees. They're not ready for your jelly anyway, and if you're going to be dropping mad cash, i.e., the annual dues of three dollars, go spend it somewhere else where your moxy is appreciated. Plus, why would you want to be part of a group of grown women who need each other's change?

The First Rule of Fight Club

Your desire to spread your wings beyond you and your fellowship doesn't mean your gal pals should take your wandering eye for outside companionship as a slight against them or allow the influx of strange women into your life to scare them. Sure, maybe the Mommy Group is just another way for moms to further blackball people from the already highly exclusive female social group that is Motherhood, but when Allison told Jillian she was dipping a toe in this pool, Jillian said, "DO IT" (and wanted to know if there was any chance she could sit in and take minutes). Nothing is going to endanger the bond we share with our soul sisters, whether you're a new mother or not. Besides, *friendship* isn't really the right word we would use to describe the majority of relationships formed within the rigid confines of the Mommy Group. And can they ever be rigid.

Immediately upon signing up, you may be made familiar with their "chartered rules" and "guidelines." Nothing says, "welcoming and relaxed" like a strict set of dos and don'ts. In the world of Mommy Groups, where there are laws in place, there are laws to be enforced. But wait a minute, aren't we all meant to be grown-ups? Aren't moms tangible proof of just that? Why is everyone having these mini-peeps if they can't come out of the pregnancy experience with unconditional adult status? Well, adults or not, you can't have a mom around without having to be made aware of a few ground rules. Moms and rules are in it to win it. Moms and rules have each others' backs. If you screw with the moms, the rules will get you. If you screw with the rules, the moms will get you. There's Batman and Robin, and then there are moms and rules. They are the original dynamic duo.

Though the group-to-group specifics may vary, the main criteria moms want to regulate is the level of commitment. It is not uncommon for there to be a designated number of permitted "no shows" within a six-month period before a member is subject to removal. If you are a habitual bailer like most of our gender, consider yourself already discharged. Moms also revisit your standard "play nice" rules, such as "Don't judge each other," "Don't impose your parenting styles on someone else," and "Don't let yourself or your child kick anyone's ass" (this can prove to be the toughest one to follow, it's been said). It almost feels as if the moms are placing too many constraints on the experience, which can end up sucking the joy out of the whole gregarious affair. But really, what can anyone expect? Sucking away joy isn't just in a mother's wheelhouse; it is the wheelhouse. In fact, we remember our very own mothers sucking most of the joy straight out of the complete duration of high school (the "joy vacuum years," as Jillian later referred to them in one of her highly dramatized LiveJournal entries). Of course, now when we look back through our thirty-three-year-old perspectives, we realize they were pretty on point with every decision they made. We can already feel one giant "I told you so" coming both our ways . . .

If you plan on signing up for the long haul, make sure you adhere to the group's constitution with minimal questions asked. Bending and/or breaking rules can lead to expulsion (yes, expulsion), and if you lose access, your friends lose their vicarious access, too, and that's not fun for anybody.

Online Forums

Maybe you aren't too hot about the ride-or-die commitment that is expected or having strange noses poking around in your personal business. Mommy groups aren't all that bad, even the ones that are. But if you find that they are stressing you out and that you're feeling pigeonholed to act a certain way, dress a certain way, or just project a persona that is getting too far away from your own, you don't need to stay. Instead, why not introduce yourself to the world of online parenting forums? Thanks to the Internet, you can lap up all the Mommy Group hijinks while maintaining complete anonymity (should you desire), thereby avoiding the forced participation of park dates and potlucks. Even you, the black sheep of the parenting world, will have an opportunity to tap in and out of the craziness at the click of a mouse, totally undetected. All the juicy truths women are too afraid to say in their real-life groups are being said here, and, luckily for you and your besties, they are spreading across every inner crevice and outer edge of the world wide web with the virulence of a frosh-week chlamydia outbreak. This makes finding a forum worth following a breeze—and getting hooked should take even less time.

If you take this route, you won't be sentenced to any weekly or bi-weekly engagements. You can sit on the couch, in your very own living room, and yuk it up with us behind your laptop. For the days when you're feeling brazen, you can always dive in with your own two cents. There is nothing wrong with wanting to get a piece of the action now and then or stir a pot begging to be stirred. However, if you are going to act as a part-time contributor, there are a few ropes you need to learn.

Adopt the Lingo

One thing a lot of women tend to forget to do when entering unknown territory is become well-versed in the language of their new community. When Allison moved to Holland, she made sure to master a few keys phrases like "Where's the bathroom?" "Is it multiple or single stalls?" and "What are the acoustics like?" You know, the basics.

Thing is, it's hard to chit-chat when nobody knows what you're trying to say. That's why the smart-ass parents of the virtual world have composed a glossary of acronyms giving mothers (and fathers!) a way to communicate using fewer letters expressed in their favorite font in ALL CAPS. As far as we can tell, there are approximately ninety-nine in operation and only two reasons we can think of as to why an online code was created to fill in for their offline yelling:

1. Acting as a crutch for Mom Brain,
2. or allowing mothers to satisfy the inherent desire to be succinct (despite their defining inability).

We're all aware how bad moms are about being concise with language. It's one of those things that worsens with age. Think about all the verbal exchanges you've shared over the years with your mom on the phone. How many times, out of every time, do you hang up confident that a) the call was necessary, and b) you understood exactly what she was talking about? We're guessing not many, but god bless 'em for thinking that a couple of acronyms could make up for all the loose ends we're left with whenever they neglect to explain or tie up their side of the conversation.

In all fairness, if mommy shorthand works for you, then let mommy shorthand work for you. Imagine your delight when you shave *seconds* off the usual handful of minutes it takes for you to create a thread or write a response in your favorite forum—and simply by incorporating a few individual letters instead of actual words. The complete list can be found on Jezebel.com in an article called "An Overwhelming Glossary of Mommy Message Board Lingo" by Tracie Egan Morrissey. Here are the ten we feel you should familiarize yourself with, not necessarily based on relevance but more on their *"seriously?"* factor.

1. AIH: Artificial insemination with husband's sperm
2. AIO: All-in-one; this means you don't need a separate cover over a disposable diaper
3. BFN: Big fat negative (as in a pregnancy test)
4. DXP: Dear ex-partner, for people who are still on good terms with their exes
5. GD: Gestational diabetes
6. LAM: Lactational amenorrhea method; referring to natural infertility while breastfeeding
7. MC: Miscarriage
8. OPK: Ovulation predictor test kit
9. POF: Premature ovarian failure
10. VBAC: Vaginal birth after caesarean

Yes, there is apparently nothing crass about using an acronym when discussing your own miscarriage (MC) or premature ovarian failure (POF). Now if only some of these moms could figure out a way to abbreviate the birth story, we might really be getting somewhere. Anybody would take that status update, slammed with just thirty or fifty letters in a row, *in caps*, over having to see another slippery umbilical cord flash across their screen any day.

Not Everything Is for Everybody

It takes courage just to try one of these groups on for size, and if it doesn't fit there is no need to wait for your honorable (or dishonorable) discharge. It's not like you've enrolled in the military, at least not technically. Best-case scenario: you end up finding what you're looking for; worst-case scenario: you decide to back out and, because of social politics, are forced to play fugitive in your own neighborhood. It's no big deal, but you might want to find someone to run your errands and play damage control while in hiding. Embracing agoraphobia as you wait for either the gossip train to slow down or for someone to overshadow your scandal with an even meatier one of their own is a game we are very familiar with (Allison was essentially Jillian's overworked publicist between the ages of eighteen to twenty-two). Once the heat is over, you can slip back into the daily grind with little attention paid to your recent disbandment. Stick it out or stick it to 'em; whichever way you're leaning toward, you'll never miss out. There's always a virtual world willing to accept you anytime, from anywhere, and in any pair of sweats you choose.

ABOUT FACEBOOK . . .

There is an elephant in the room, and you're probably wondering how the flip we've managed to miss it. We haven't; we know an elephant when we see one. We *know* Facebook is a huge part of the problem with mothers-to-be and the mothers-that-be. We know that a lot of their social media behavior is in desperate need of an intervention, but we also know that if said intervention were to go from a hypothetical situation to an organized sting, none of those claiming to take offense would have the balls to show up, especially if the subject is someone they hold dear. That's just the way it is, because for every mom out there, unwittingly overdosing their social circles on photos of their kids or statuses about how bright so-and-so is for their age and how much television they *don't* watch, there are at least five friends who will never ever call them out on it.

You've got to hand it to your OG's—it isn't easy scrolling past the fifth installment of your "April 2017" album series or, as everyone else will refer to it, "calculated glimpses into the family life you hope people believe you lead." We get it. You want everyone to see how often you play outdoors with your children, like a good mother. You project someone who is happy and proud, that is clear; but equally evident is a mother who is scared she's not doing enough and is in constant pursuit of (feigned or sincere) recognition. Just like the rest of us on Facebook.

Everyone understands, and, most important, nobody cares either way. And that's a *good* thing. You can relax. We're all friends here, and like we said, nobody is going to confront you to your face. It's not as easy to get after a new mom when one genuinely cares about her well-being. It's like getting mad at a puppy; puppies try so hard, but when they get overexcited they make a mess. And although some of you may not be peeing and pooping on the carpets, you still seem to have trouble controlling the shit you're spraying onto newsfeeds.

Just know that we *know*, and if anything, we wouldn't mind knowing less. So, when you're gunning it for the point of no return by deciding to go all Anne Geddes with an umbilical stump photo shoot or adding a filter to a picture of a dirty diaper, be grateful if you're met with poorly veiled misdirection from trusted pals. A simple "Dude, you can't put that on the Internet" is usually enough to put those decisions on trial, leading to a discussion that will almost always rule in favor of the plaintiff. But for the most part, when it comes to the merciless uploads and unsubstantiated bragging, friends will be left mindlessly hitting the Like button and consulting their mental collection of generalized compliments (i.e., "Aw!" "Cute!" "He's/She's so big!") before continuing with life.

Almost every chapter we've covered previously is tied into Facebook in some way or another. The pregnancy announcement, the ultrasound, the cravings, the maternity shoot, the placenta—it's all there. We could have focused solely on social media and still filled a book, but we all know how that would read. And if you are looking for a more in-depth exposé on the matter, the tell-all, *STFU, Parents: The Jaw-Dropping, Self-Indulgent, and Occasionally Rage-Inducing World of Parent Overshare* by Blair Koenig, is already up for purchase. So, if you feel cheated out of a chapter, don't fret, Ms. Koenig has got you covered.

YOU'RE STILL HERE, WE'RE STILL HERE, THINGS ARE DIFFERENT, THIS IS LIFE

Let's talk about what happens now. The entrance of a baby into your life has changed your relationships, and there will be times when it feels like things are only changing for the worse; whenever the girls are meeting up for drinks, you're meeting the deadlines of an infant's napping schedule. You'll worry they don't appreciate how much you wish you could join them, while at the same time you're just happy to finally have a legitimate reason to stay home. And even though you're no longer able to drop whatever you're doing to answer their late-night distress calls or act as the buffer in a group date every time someone swipes right on Tinder, friends *do* understand, or at least they *will* eventually. New normals are just that:

new, and getting used to them isn't always a straight shot up the y-axis. Let everyone choose their own speed as they make their way across the learning curve, because some people warm to unfamiliar dynamics faster than others, and that's okay.

That said, don't let anything or anyone diminish the magnitude of what you've been through. There's this great line in a very pregnant Ali Wong's Netflix special, *Baby Cobra*, where she rubs her stomach and talks about taking a hiatus from adult responsibilities because she's too "busy making an eyeball." That is *not* hyperbole. And then, like many of the women before her, she made elbows and antagonistic muscle systems and kidneys and all those other things that make a person a person.

Doesn't that so perfectly demonstrate the magnitude and fucked-up fantasticalness of procreation? It's a lot. *It's a freaking lot.* And after taking nine months to carefully craft a human being, you have to care for it. Care for it as if you were on an eighteen-year walk with a Fabergé egg in a spoon—but the egg is kicking and screaming and the walk turns out to be a series of successive faceplants. It's scary, and, yes, everyone is afraid of breaking the baby. Irrational fear comes for moms hard; but let's be honest, it comes for everyone. Every time Jillian gets behind the wheel of a car, she always thinks to herself,

God, I hope I don't kill somebody today (macabre, but true). Those dark-and-dreary worst-case-scenario feelings for her are situational, but for moms like you they occur every other second.

Luckily, babies get bigger. They get stronger. They become less breakable, and making it through each day without busting up your flimsy, as-durable-as-a-house-of-cards child will get easier. Thank god for the growing and fusion of bones. It gives you a chance to get emotionally situated, and the resulting all-encompassing exhale will affect everything in your path. You will become more adventurous, you will have time to listen, and you might even make an appearance at a get-together and talk behind the other guests' backs like the woman your friends all know and love. Eventually, you'll wonder how those first years got away from you when you're posting, "I don't know who cried more?" underneath a picture of your son or daughter's first day of school (another madly original contribution to the colorful tapestry that is the "First Week of September Facebook Feed") or when you're holding yourself back, like all good moms do, from telling other parents you suspect your child of being a prodigy. Because the clock is ticking, and it ticks fast.

So, good mother, be a hero on the days you feel like being a hero, and as for the other days, the days when everything shifts from "Look what I did!" to "What have I done . . . ," remember this: parenting is an incredibly serious game played best when not being taken too seriously. It's also a game that happens to pair well with wine (again with the moms and wines—when are these two going to get their own show?). Let the pregnant ones pour, and everyone else can exercise their right to sleep off a hangover. Look at you, back to business as usual.

ACKNOWLEDGMENTS

Jillian Parsons

First and foremost, I would like to thank my sister Katy, not only because I owe her dearly for playing editor-at-large when there was no editor-at-all, but also because she has, many times over, told me to do so. This manuscript may never have been picked up if it wasn't for her tweaks and suggestions throughout the embryonic stages . . . is something I am sure she would want me to clarify for the audience. Lucky for her I have, and lucky for me, it's true.

To my contributor extraordinaire, Allison Baerken, whom I love and respect beyond expression, who came on board just when we thought everything was sinking, and who had the balls to get behind almost every word between these pages (though she remains staunchly against any mention of "anal"). She has given me her stories—disgusting and humiliating—enabling me to elevate the points and hard-land the punchlines. Private moments are not something she discloses lightly, so to you, Allison, I am forever indebted (which, as we both know, is nothing new—at least not in monetary terms).

On behalf of her and I, we would like to thank Priya Doraswamy and Lotus Lane Literary for taking this unlikely project under their wing, along with our editor, Kim Lim, and Skyhorse Publishing, for seeing the merit in our voice. Moms are a tough sell and our angle was an objectively risky one—we are grateful to have you on our team and to be part of yours.

To our families—thank you for the unconditional and at times uninformed support (it's been up for pre-sale since *October*, Mom, *stop asking*). May this book's success strike the perfect balance of reverence and jealousy in our siblings and an unwavering sense of enthusiastic worship among our parents. To our friends, the ones with kids and the ones without, your abilities to be made fun of are admirable and your abilities to make fun of others are something we should probably sit down and address. Thank you for spilling your guts and letting us publish them, for bringing the beer when things looked grim, and for bringing some more when things looked up.

Lastly, to everyone we love, thank you for the continued encouragement—through every recreation of this adventure and beyond. We cannot imagine a comparable way to repay you, but know it will not be with a free book. We are not made of money or paperbacks. It's full price all 'round. Sorry.